Perinatal Asphyxia

Perinatal Asphyxia

Alberto Lacoius-Petruccelli, M.D.

Cornell University School of Medicine
New York, New York

Plenum Medical Book Company • New York and London

Library of Congress Cataloging in Publication Data

Lacoius-Petruccelli, Alberto.
  Perinatal asphyxia.

  Bibliography: p.
  Includes index.
  1. Aphyxia Neonatorum. I. Title. [DNLM: 1. Asphyxia Neonatorum. 2. Fetal Anoxia.
WQ 450 L142p]
RJ256.L33   1986   618.92'2   86-25176
ISBN-13: 978-1-4612-9011-7   e-ISBN-13: 978-1-4613-1807-1
DOI: 10.1007/ 978-1-4613-1807-1

© 1987 Plenum Publishing Corporation
Softcover reprint of the hardcover 1st edition 1987
233 Spring Street, New York, N.Y. 10013

Plenum Medical Book Company is an imprint of Plenum Publishing Corporation

DEDICATED TO:

Dr. Roberto Caldeyro-Barcia,
Director of the Latin-American Center
for Perinatology in Montevideo, Uruguay,
pioneer of perinatology,
maestro of neonatologists,
with admiration and respect

Dr. Peter Auld, Director of the
Perinatology Center, New York Hospital,
for giving me an opportunity to learn
about perinatology,
with gratitude

Dr. Mary Allen Engle,
Professor of Pediatric Cardiology and
Director of Pediatric Cardiology,
New York Hospital–
Cornell University Medical College,
with appreciation for her advice in
the preparation of this manuscript

Dr. Rosa Lee Nemir, Professor of
Pediatrics, New York University, for
her kindness and wise suggestions in
the preparation of this work

Preface

The aim of this book is to transmit the message that asphyxia is the major cause of infant mortality in the neonatal period. The sequelae of asphyxia—if severe, causing cerebral palsy; if mild, leading to MBD to seizures— are all potential risks.

It is important to make young physicians and nurses aware of this complication of the birth period, how to avoid it, and how to treat it. Facilitating such awareness is the chief purpose of this book.

Alberto Lacoius-Petruccelli

New York

Contents

1

Asphyxia
Definitions, History, and Incidence

> *Stage of depression in the newborn*
> *often following a difficult delivery*
> —William Little

Definitions

Lack of adequate oxygenation is called asphyxia; lack of adequate blood supply is called ischemia. Both are important causes of brain damage and death and affect babies during intrauterine life, labor, and delivery and shortly after birth.

For the adequate-for-gestational-age (AGA) newborn offspring of a normal pregnancy with Apgar score of 9/10, life prognosis is good. Complicated pregnancies involving very-low-birth-weight (VLBW) babies, those small for gestational age (SGA), intrauterine growth retardation (IUGR), and difficult deliveries are frequent causes of low Apgar scores, which are an expression of

11

asphyxia. For the high-risk pregnancy (HRP) giving birth to a VLBW, IUGR, or SGA baby with Apgar scores under 5, perinatal death is a risk; with Apgar scores of 7, neurological sequelae such as cerebral palsy (CP) and seizures are risks and may become apparent later in life.

CP is a brain dysfunction characterized by a nonprogressive disorder arising from maldevelopment of the brain occurring during intrauterine life or at birth. Sensory and motor dysfunction, spasticity, delayed milestones, persistence of primitive reflexes, and association with cognitive deficits, seizures, and speech and vision defects are elements observed in this syndrome.

Seizures are paroxysmal episodes of involuntary movements, either generalized or affecting specific groups of muscles, with or without loss of consciousness.

Both CP and seizures are expressions of moderate to severe asphyxial stress at birth.

History

The pioneer figure in the study of birth asphyxia was Dr. William Little, a British orthopedic surgeon, who, in 1861, first connected abnormal deliveries and birth trauma with neurological damage. Presenting his observations of 20 years, he related birth asphyxia to newborn deaths and to different types of neurological sequelae that developed as the child grew older. He also described different types of spastic paresis and retardation.

Mathison, in 1910, was able to relate asphyxia and bradycardia. In 1928, Schmidt reported the relationship between newborn asphyxia and hypercarbia, metabolic acidosis, and depression of the respiratory center, which left the cells of the CNS unable to utilize oxygen later on.

In 1930, Eastman defined asphyxia as the inability of the newborn to breathe, showing apnea to be related to a deficient oxygen supply during the period of labor. His investigations identified hypoxia and hypercapnia as factors responsible for the initiation of respiration at birth. He was able to measure oxygen saturation in the umbilical vein and lactate in cord blood and documented the absence of signs of trauma or bleeding in cases of death resulting from birth asphyxia. He demonstrated that metabolic lactic acidosis occurs in cases of severe asphyxia in newborns.

Eastman also investigated the role of anesthesia given to the mother in producing depression and apnea in the newborn.

In 1953, Dr. Virginia Apgar defined the Apgar score and showed the relationship between birth asphyxia and low Apgar scores.

Meyer and Windle, in 1964, demonstrated that hypoxia and hypercapnia led to cellular damage and brain lesions and that anoxia caused brain edema and permeability changes, which can lead to ischemia and a reduction in cardiac output.

Caldeyro-Barcia of Uruguay, in 1960, developed the technique of fetal monitoring, which enabled him to demonstrate stages of intrauterine asphyxia as determined by fetal scalp oxygen measurements. He then studied the degrees of fetal compromise as associated with early (type I), late (type II), and variable (type III) fetal decelerations. He also described the relationship between birth asphyxia as reflected in fetal decelerations and neurological sequelae later in life.

Caldeyro-Barcia also determined intraamniotic pressure, which led to a new understanding of the forces involved in labor.

Thus, in just a century, remarkable progress has been made in understanding the causes of birth asphyxia, its prophylaxis, methods of documentation, and approaches to treating the asphyxiated newborn. Improved knowledge of the pathophysiology of asphyxial stress and better equipment and trained personnel in perinatology centers have led to a reduction in neonatal mortality among high-risk infants from 80% to 10%.

Incidence

As many as 10% of births may be affected by asphyxia. Statistically, one baby with CP is born every hour in the United States (8760 new cases per year). One baby with minor neurological damage or minimal brain dysfunction (MBD) is born every 5 min (105,120 new cases every year).

Nearly 4 million babies are born each year in the United States; 3% of them die. This means that 120,000 infant deaths occur in the first year. Of these, 75% occur in the first month of life, the neonatal period, and the majority of these are among "high-risk" babies who are small at birth:

1. Preterm babies less than 37 weeks of gestation.
2. Premature babies less than 35 weeks of gestation.
3. Postterm babies more than 42 weeks of gestation.
4. Complicated full-term pregnancies (37–42 weeks).

The cause of death in this group is most often brain asphyxia or hemorrhage or immaturity of lungs or other major systems. Thus, asphyxia and hemorrhage represent the major causes of death in the newborn period.

These may be less severe in some cases and permit the baby to survive, but residual effects may be seen later in life as the child develops. This would explain cases of cerebral palsy as well as learning disabilities and seizures.

New advances in technology, particularly in perinatology, offer hope. Perinatology is the specialty in medicine that focuses on the baby from 26 weeks of intrauterine life to the end of the perinatal period (first 4 weeks of life after birth).

Progress has been made in the early diagnosis of complicated, high-risk pregnancies, which produce high-risk babies, and early treatment of those pregnancies and early care of these babies in neonatal intensive care units (perinatology centers) or tertiary care centers in the last 10 years have made possible the recovery of these infants. However, much remains to be done to improve the quality of life of these children as they grow older.

2

Occurrence *in Utero*, at Birth, and after Delivery

The cause of death from asphyxia is explained as a lack of oxygenation or insufficient oxygenation (hypoxia). If the asphyxia is prolonged and there is an inadequate blood supply to major organs, particularly the brain (ischemia), causing lesions in the brain and/or brain hemorrhage, then the baby affected by asphyxia is at particular risk. This can occur in intrauterine life, at the time of delivery, or shortly after delivery, affecting the newborn baby.

Asphyxia in Intrauterine Life

In this group, asphyxia is an expression of lack of oxygenation of the baby *in utero* whose mother's health is complicated by seizures, drugs, alcohol, infections, and toxemia or eclampsia. This complication will affect the third trimester of pregnancy and represents a placental dysfunction. There can sometimes be hypertension, edema, and/or seizures (eclampsia). These conditions may endanger the baby by compromising the blood and oxygen supply of the fetus and causing intrauterine asphyxia.

Asphyxia at the Time of Delivery

This second form of asphyxia arises from obstetric complications that create asphyxia at the time of delivery and affect the uterus, placenta, and/or labor itself. Among obstetric complications, the following may be causes of asphyxia:

1. Cord around the neck, which may cause asphyxia by compression of the umbilical vein.
2. Contractions of the uterus or dystocias of contractions.
3. Cephalopelvic disproportion caused by a mismatch in size between the fetus and the pelvis of the mother, which may create mechanical compressions and lead to asphyxia.
4. Placenta previa, which is a placenta implanted in the lower part of the uterus, may cause significant bleeding at the time of labor and may also lead to asphyxia.
5. Abruptio placenta, in which the placenta separates before the baby is born, can cause severe bleeding and asphyxia.
6. Fast or precipitated deliveries, which can adversely affect the baby's adjustment mechanism as well as abruptly compressing the umbilical cord, may also cause asphyxia.

7. Early rupture of membranes, either induced or spontaneous, more than 24 hr before delivery can cause infection and asphyxia.

Asphyxia after Delivery

This group presents after the baby is born in asphyxial stress; it is particularly important when it affects small babies, premature infants (<35 weeks of gestation), and postmature babies (>42 weeks of gestation). Among babies less than 35 weeks of gestation, who have immature systems and are susceptible to asphyxia, and those over 42 weeks of gestation, who are subject to asphyxia from placental dysfunction, there can be fetal distress, meconium aspiration, and infection at the time of delivery.

The respiratory distress syndrome (RDS) affects small premature babies with immature lungs (hyaline membrane disease, HMD) and can be a cause of asphyxia as a result of inadequate pulmonary gas exchange or ventilation. The RDS can also affect the postmature infant who, because of hypoxic stress from placental insufficiency, may become asphyxial *in utero*. The passing and aspiration of meconium will create a severe condition of congested lungs and asphyxia referred to as the syndrome of meconium aspiration.

Other causes of asphyxia after birth include hematologic factors such as hemolytic disease of the newborn, causing severe anemia and leading to poor oxygen transport. This condition is known as anemic anoxia.

3

Physiopathology of Asphyxia and Its Staging

Brain changes occur in the newborn suffering insufficient blood oxygenation at birth. Inadequate oxygenation of the brain may cause different types of lesions, depending on the nature and duration of the stress as well as the degree of maturity of the fetus. If anoxia affects babies 37 weeks or older, lesions caused by asphyxia will be observed in the cortex or subcortical area of the brain. In premature babies, asphyxia may create lesions in the periventricular area and the matrix. Interestingly, the immature brain is more resistant to asphyxia than the adult brain, but the reason for this difference is unknown.

Inadequate oxygenation and insufficient blood flow at birth can affect the transition from oxygenation via the umbilical vein of the placenta to oxygenation from the expanding lungs. The clamping and cutting of the umbilical cord at birth stimulate the expansion of the lungs and diminish pulmonary vascular resistance; this favors blood flow to the lungs and expansion of the alveoli. At this point, the process of pulmonary respiration starts. Increased blood flow to the pulmonary vein increases the flow of blood to the left atrium and left ventricle and favors closure of the PDA and foramen ovale. From this time on, systemic pressure is higher than venous pressure, establishing a left-to-right shunt, and the closing of this shunt characterizes the normal pattern of circulation and oxygenation of the newborn.

This normal pattern of oxygenation that starts at birth, the transition from placental to pulmonary oxygenation from the expanding lungs, requires a perfect and rapid adjustment to avoid asphyxia and ischemia (poor blood flow). In this process of adjustment, there are three stages of hypoxia.

Stage 1 Hypoxia

Insufficient oxygen supply stimulates the stress mechanisms, epinephrine release, and a shift in blood supply from peripheral organs (limbs, GI system, skin) to major organs (brain, heart, and adrenals). This guarantees an adequate blood supply to essential organs such as brain and heart.

Clinically, in stage 1 hypoxia the newborn infant still looks active, and his color is pink with only mild distal cyanosis; the infant has good to low muscle tone and has normal reflexes.

Neurologically, pupils become dilated (an expression of hypoxic stress), and there are no seizures. The heart is accelerated. At this point, the mild hypoxic condition is reflected in minimal neurological compromise, low tone, or jitters; the lack of oxygen is not severe; and EEG is normal. If there is no improvement in the oxygenation of the baby, or the condition does not respond to treatment, then asphyxia progresses. The systemic blood pressure, which was normal during the first stage of the reaction, starts to decline as a defense mechanism (reaction to hypoxic stress); the pulse, which had first accelerated, starts to slow down to bradycardia. Therefore, hypoxia progresses to stage 2.

Stage 2 Hypoxia

At this stage there is progressive bradycardia and hypotension, and the blood flow to vital organs diminishes; ischemia then complicates hypoxia. Stasis of blood follows, particularly in the brain, and this creates congestion, increases capillary permeability, and leads to the swelling or edema of brain tissue (cerebral edema), which produces an increase in intracranial pressure.

Stage 3 Hypoxia

Hypoxia is reflected in metabolic changes, retention of CO_2 (hypercapnia), lactic acid accumulation, metabolic acidosis, and low HCO_3, resulting in both respiratory and metabolic acidosis. This stage is also characterized by cerebral edema, increased intracranial pressure, hypoxia complicated by ischemia, and cerebral metabolic acidosis. There is progressive brain asphyxia.

Clinically, lethargy, low muscle tone to total muscle relaxation (severe hypotonia), lack of reflexes, and poor sucking reflexes are observed. The pupils, which were dilated, constrict, the heart slows down (bradycardia), blood pressure drops, and seizures can be seen; the EEG shows a low voltage threshold for seizure activity.

At this level, if the baby is adequately treated, survival can be possible. However, the brain lesions related to asphyxia, ischemia, and metabolic acidosis will result in neurological sequelae or other residual effects of severe brain asphyxia. If there is no adequate treatment, the progressive and irreversible asphyxia will be reflected in a baby whose condition deteriorates from lethargy to coma; areflexia, fixed pupils, low EEG voltage, seizures (rarely), total muscle relaxation, extreme bradycardia, and periods of apnea and periodic breathing are seen. At this stage, death is the final event.

4

Work-up and Treatment in the Newborn

Delivery Room, Nursery, and Perinatal ICU

Work-up Required for a Baby with Respiratory Distress

The premature infant with RDS requires continuous evaluation of its respiratory status as determined by arterial blood gas (ABG) measurements to make possible appropriate adjustments of ventilator pressures, FiO_2, rates, and I/E ratios and to determine when it is appropriate to switch from intermittent positive-pressure breathing (IPPB) to continuous positive airway pressure (CPAP).

The respiratory work-up includes, in addition, chest X rays to document progress and to determine the severity of hyaline membrane disease (HMD) or of complications such as atelectasis and pneumothorax.

The results of the work-up of a newborn with RDS will indicate the degree of respiratory compromise: low pH and low PO_2 indicate poor oxygen saturation; high PCO_2 indicates poor CO_2 exchange; and low HCO_3 implies the presence of metabolic acidosis such as that seen in severely asphyxiated babies.

In order to determine the degree of compromise in RDS and to direct appropriate treatment, the work-up must include metabolic evaluation as well as hematologic, neurological, infectious disease, cardiovascular, and renal testing.

Metabolic

Metabolic evaluation requires measurement of electrolytes: Na^+, Cl^-, K^+, and HCO_3. In babies with severe asphyxia and metabolic changes, it is necessary to determine Ca^{2+} and glucose levels, BUN, and serum creatinine, which reflect the degree of renal involvement; babies under severe asphyxial stress may have low glucose, low calcium, high BUN, and high creatinine.

Hematologic

A blood count including a differential and platelet count is needed if there is anemia or infection.

Neurological

For the severely asphyxiated infant, including one in a coma, the neurological work-up should include skull X rays, TORCH titers in SGA infants or those with small heads, and sonography and CAT scan to determine types and locations of lesions. If there is risk of infection, the work-up should also include blood, urine, and CSF cultures for identification of pathogens and sensitivity testing.

Renal

The renal work-up should include electrolytes, BUN, and creatinine levels.

General Procedures

If the newborn infant does not breathe within the first 30 sec, the baby is suctioned to remove secretions, given oxygen, stimulated, and kept warm. If the baby does not respond within the next 30–60 sec, it is "bagged": a mask is applied over the nose and mouth, and oxygen (up to 100%) is given by push at a frequency of 30–40/min.

If the baby does not respond to this procedure within 2–3 min, then it should be intubated, which involves the introduction of a polyethylene tube (2.5–3.5 mm in diameter) through the nose (nasal intubation), throat, and larynx to the trachea using a Miller laryngoscope (#1 or #2). This is an emergency procedure to provide oxygen and pressure to distend the lungs; it is used only for babies who are born asphyxiated and do not breathe for 2–2.5 min and serves to correct apnea of the newborn, which, if untreated, would lead to brain asphyxia.

At 3 min, if the baby shows gasping and a heart rate that is < 100 beats/min (bradycardia) and irregular, 100%

oxygen is given via the endotracheal tube, epinephrine (1:10,000) is administered (0.1 mg/kg i.v. plus some via the endotracheal tube), and cardiac massage is begun.

After several minutes, if the intubated baby shows irregular breathing, a heart rate of < 100 beats/min, and arterial blood gases characteristic of metabolic acidosis ($\downarrow$pH, $\downarrow$PO$_2$, $\downarrow$HCO$\bar{3}$) or respiratory acidosis ($\downarrow$pH, $\uparrow$PCO$_2$, $\downarrow$PO$_2$), then NaHCO$_3$ is given (1–2 mEq/kg slowly i.v., by umbilical vein if that is catheterized).

If poor perfusion is present (weak pulses, tachycardia, distal cyanosis), then albumin (5%, 10 ml/kg slow push) and calcium gluconate (10%, 2 ml/kg) are given.

If the baby develops symptoms of persistent fetal circulation (PFC) and blood gases show respiratory acidosis, then treatment consists of 100% oxygen with assisted ventilation (IPPB at pressures of 35/5 cm H$_2$O, 30–60 breaths/min) and pancuronium (Pavulon®) to produce muscle relaxation.

If the baby shows signs of heart failure (decreased blood pressure and heart rate, ECG signs, and appearance on chest X ray), dopamine (2–20 mg/kg per min i.v.) is added.

If renal failure is present (output < 1 ml/kg per hr), the intravenous fluids should be reduced to half maintenance: 35–50 ml/kg per hr plus output.

If electrolyte studies show low serum calcium (< 5–6 mg/dl), 10% calcium gluconate is added (2 ml/kg i.v. by push) with control of pulse.

In the small premature newborn weighing < 1500 g, necrotizing enterocolitis (NEC) must be considered if guaiac-positive stools and abdominal distension are present with characteristic abdominal X-ray findings. Oral feedings should be withheld until the gastrointestinal system has stabilized. If there are signs of bleeding ($\downarrow$Hb, $\downarrow$Hct, $\uparrow$PT/PTT, $\downarrow$platelet count), then blood or platelet transfusions are indicated. If respiration and color improve; heart rate is approximately 100 beats/min; pulse, respiration, temperature, and blood pressure are stable; chest X ray shows lungs expanding normally; and blood glucose is 30–45 mg/dl, then dextrose (10%, 2 ml/kg) is added to the i.v. If there is a slow pulse and blood pressure is below 40 mm Hg, volume expanders such as 5% albumin are given at 10 ml/kg and repeated in 30 min if needed.

If apnea develops or RDS is present, assisted ventilation (IPPB) is started in an attempt to achieve blood gas control: pH 7.35–7.45, P_{CO_2} 35–45 mm Hg, P_{O_2} 80–100 mm Hg. The IPPB is started with pressures of 35/5 cm H_2O, FiO_2 25–100%, rate 30–60 breaths/min, I/E ratio 1:2.

If metabolic acidosis complicates respiratory acidosis with pH < 7.2, P_{O_2} < 30 mm Hg, and HCO_3^- < 8–10 mM, then $NaHCO_3$, 1 mEq/kg, is added to correct the base deficit. Base deficit is calculated as:

$$(20 - [HCO_3^-]) \times 0.4 \times \text{body weight}$$

and half should be given by slow i.v. push. If convulsions develop, a loading dose of phenobarbital, 10 mg/kg, is added i.v., and phenobarbital blood levels are monitored for control.

If the baby has arterial P_{O_2} < 30 mm Hg, P_{CO_2} > 55–60 mm Hg, and pH < 7.3 despite 100% oxygen and is not breathing spontaneously, he is in respiratory acidosis and requires assisted ventilation.

5

Mechanical Ventilators

Mechanical ventilators (Fig. 1) are designed to help babies with respiratory distress. The objective is to improve exchange and to treat respiratory insufficiency.

Respiratory distress syndrome (RDS) caused by hyaline membrane disease (HMD) is the main cause of infant mortality affecting prematures in the neonatal period. However, death from HMD in the premature infant has been significantly reduced from 80% to 10% since the early 1970s, and the use of mechanical ventilators has been the main contributing factor. Better understanding of the physiopathology of the premature infant, better equipment, the creation of tertiary care centers for the better care of high-risk infants (HRI), and the preparation of more skillful personnel explain this development.

The use of mechanical ventilators is, however, not without risks. Bronchopulmonary dysplasia (BPD) could be a late complication related to the use of mechanical ventilators, since pneumothorax is a possible complica-

tion in the acute stage. Central nervous system hemorrhage and intraventricular hemorrhage (IVH) are complications in the very-low-birth-weight (VLBW) baby who
develops RDS because of HMD and requires treatment
with ventilators.

Indications for the Use of Mechanical Ventilators

In the premature infant with RDS, respiratory failure can be clinically documented by the following: (1)
progressive tachypnea (more than 80/min), (2) marked
intercostal and subcostal retractions, (3) cyanosis, and (4)
apnea. The laboratory work-up, including arterial blood
gases (ABG), shows a rising PCO_2 (60 mm Hg), a low
PO_2 (<50 mm Hg in 100% O_2), and a low pH (<7.25).
This indicates hypoxemia leading to respiratory acidosis
(hypoxia with hypercapnia) and reflects lung disease.
There is increased pulmonary vascular resistance, increased central nervous system (CNS) pressure, and
diminished cardiac output. This is the clinical presentation in a premature or, in particular, in the VLBW that
indicates respiratory failure and justifies the use of
mechanical ventilators.

There are two types of positive-pressure mechanical
ventilators: volume ventilators and pressure ventilators.

The volume ventilator delivers unchanged tidal volume (volume of gas inhaled or exhaled during a normal
respiratory cycle, typically 7–10 ml/kg).

Pressure ventilators deliver a volume of air that
changes on each inspiration to a set inspiratory pressure.
In a case of progressive RDS with developing atelectasis, volume respirators do not help because delivered
pressures do not change. Instead, pressure ventilators

may resolve the progressive atelectasis by increasing the peak inspiratory pressure (PIP) to 30–35 cm H_2O, by changing the post-end-expiratory pressure (PEEP), or by changing the relationship of PIP to PEEP.

The pressure ventilator may operate as a controlled ventilator or as an assisted ventilator. As a controlled ventilator, each inspiration is initiated by the ventilator, and respirations are totally under the control of the ventilator. As an assisted ventilator, the inspiratory effort triggers the ventilator.

How to Operate the Pressure Ventilator

A classical mechanical positive-pressure ventilator is the Bourns Model BP200 (Fig. 1). Its controls show the following:

1. Pressures: PIP/PEEP. Peak inspiratory pressure usually is set at 30–35 cm H_2O. Higher values may create a risk of elevating pulmonary venous pressure and compromising the cardiac output. Post-end-expiratory pressure usually is set at 5 cm H_2O. Too low a PEEP may favor atelectasis.
2. Oxygen. The FiO_2 (inspired O_2 concentration) reflects the amount of oxygen. Starting FiO_2 is usually set at 50–75% or more O_2 depending on the amount of respiratory distress and the amount of respiratory acidosis reflected by the arterial blood gases.
3. Breathing rate. This dial shows rates from 1 to 60 breaths/min. Slow rates may require higher PIP and may be used for weaning; they may raise oxygenation. Higher rates may allow a low PIP

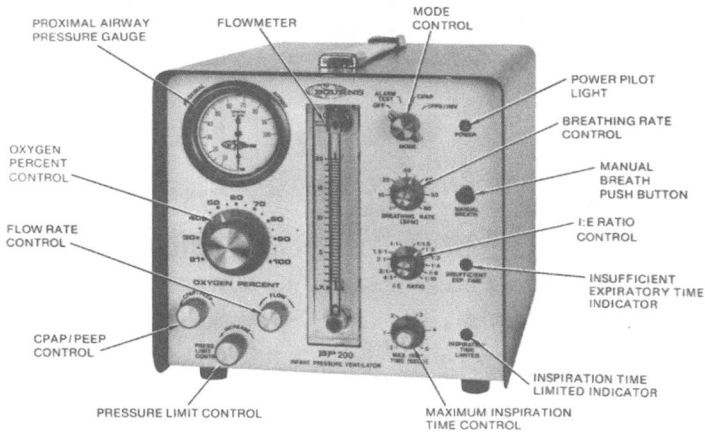

FIGURE 1. Infant pressure ventilator, Bourns model BP200, front view.

and may be indicated in persistent fetal circulation. They favor respiratory alkalosis and may
prevent atelectasis.

4. I/E ratio. This is the relationship between the du-
rations of inspiration and expiration. The dial indicates ratios from 1:1 to 1:10. In severe cases of
RDS, an I/E ratio of 2:1 may favor pulmonary
hypertension and deteriorating ABG. An I/E ratio of 1:2 is indicated, when oxygenation is no
longer a problem, to stimulate compliance, the
distensibility of the lung or chest wall as change
in volume per unit change in pressure.

5. Tidal volume. This is the volume of gas inhaled
or exhaled during a normal respiratory cycle; normal is 7–10 ml/kg. The dial of the respirator indicates CPAP/PEEP. Continuous positive airway
pressure is used when the baby starts to breathe
on his own and therefore only needs pressure to
keep the airway open. Positive end-expiratory
pressure applies pressure at the end of the expiration to maintain the alveoli open and to avoid
collapse.

6

Prognosis

The prognosis will depend on the type of asphyxia the baby presents (Tables 1–8, Figs. 2 and 3).

Stage 1 Asphyxia

If the baby is not breathing for 30 sec, he is stimulated, suctioned, and given oxygen. After this period of time the baby reacts; he will start breathing, change color from pale or cyanotic to pink, recover muscle tone, and react to oxygen stimulation.

This infant has shown an Apgar score of 5 in the first minute and reached Apgar 8/9 after the first 5 min. This baby may have a good prognosis and a good future.

Stage 2 Asphyxia

This baby represents a prolonged period of asphyxia and requires bagging and oxygen for several minutes. If

TABLE 1. Stages of Asphyxia at Birth

	Stage I (mild)	Stage II (moderate)	Stage III (severe)
Respiration	Tachypnea Retraction	Tachypnea Retraction Cyanosis	Cardiorespiratory arrhythmia Bradypnea A&B, gasping
Heart	Tachycardia	Tachycardia Arrhythmia	Bradycardia
Neurological	Active	Less active Low tone	Flaccid Seizures Coma
Blood	$\downarrow Po_2$	$\downarrow Po_2$, $\uparrow CO_2$	$\downarrow Po_2$, $\uparrow CO_2$, $\downarrow pH$
Physiopathology	Low placental blood flow Lung not expanding	Increased pulmonary vascular resistance Persistent fetal circulation	Brain asphyxia Brain hemorrhage

TABLE 2. Asphyxia in the Delivery Room

Time	Clinical findings	Treatment
1 min	Apnea Heart rate < 100 Cyanosis Flaccidity	DeLee suction Wall suction O_2 mask
2 min	Same	Bagging, 100% O_2
2–3 min	Same	Intubation with 100% O_2 Laryngoscope tube
3 min	Gasping Heart rate < 100, irregular Heart rate < 60	Intubation with 100% O_2 Epinephrine, 1:10,000, 0.1 mg/kg i.v. + ETT Cardiac massage
Several minutes	Irregular breathing Heart rate < 100 Heart rate < 60	$NaHCO_3$ for metabolic acidosis Ventilation

TABLE 3. Asphyxia in the Delivery Room

Clinical finding	Laboratory finding	Treatment
Bradycardia		Albumin, 5%, 10 ml/kg
Weak pulses		Calcium gluconate, 10%, 2 ml/kg
Persistent fetal circulation	Respiratory acidosis, low pH, high P_{CO_2}	Oxygen, IPPB Pancuronium
Heart failure	Decreased blood pressure, heart rate Chest X rays	Dopamine, 2–20 μg/kg per min
Renal failure	Urine output < 1 ml/kg per hr	Half-maintenance: 35–50 ml + output Sodium 2–4 mEq/kg per day
Hypocalcemia	5–6 mg/dl Ca	Calcium gluconate, 10%, 2 ml/kg; 24 mg/kg per day
Necrotizing enterocolitis	Guaiac-positive stools X ray	No oral feeding until stable
Bleeding	Low Hb, Hct Low PT, PTT Platelets < 50,000	Platelet transfusions 10 ml/kg

TABLE 4. Asphyxia in the Perinatal ICU

Clinical	Monitor control	Treatment
Respiration, color improved HR >100	Vital signs, pulse, respiration, temperature, BP, ABG, electrolytes, chest X rays Glucose <45	O_2 10% D/W 2 ml/kg i.v.
Low pulse Hypoglycemia Heart, CNS damage BP <40	BP <40	Expansion: 5% albumin, 10 ml/kg Repeat PRN after 20–30 min
Shock	BP <40	Dopamine i.v. or dobutamine, 2–20 μg/kg per min
If apnea persists or RDS is present	By vital signs Pulse, respiration, temperature Color RDS	Assisted ventilation and intubation are started, trying to obtain pH 7.35–7.45; P_{CO_2} 35–45; P_{O_2} 80–100; P 35/5; Fi_{C_2} 25–100; P rate 30–60
Metabolic acidosis	pH ↓ (7.30) HCO_3 ↓ (10) Pa_{O_2} ↓ (30)	$NaHCO_3$ 1 mEq/kg 150 mEq/liter Correct base deficit ≥15 mEq/liter per mm
Severe asphyxia	Twitching Convulsions	Phenobarbital, 5–20 mg/kg

Table 5. Stages of Asphyxia in the Newborn

Clinical	Asphyxia in the newborn	Delivery room treatment
Tone (+)	Transient asphyxia	Warmer
Respiration (−)	Cold	De Lee suction
Color (−)	Distal cyanosis	Wall suction (optional)
Heart rate (+)	Meconium (+)	
Reaction to stimuli (+)		
Apgar score 8		
Tone (+)	Mild asphyxia 0.5 to 1	Suction
Respiration (−)	min after 1.5-min in-	Oxygen mask
Color (−)	tubation	Bagging with 100% O_2
Heart rate (−)		
Response to stimuli (+)		
Apgar score 5–7		
Tone (−)	Severe asphyxia	Intubation with 100%
Respiration (−)	More than 1.5 min	O_2
Color (−)	Flaccid	Cardiac massage until
Heart rate (−)	Heart rate less than	heart rate is higher
Response to stimuli (−)	100	than 100
Apgar score 1	Apnea	

TABLE 6. Elements of Evaluation of the Asphyxial–Ischemic
Newborn at Different Gestational Ages

Finding	At 28 weeks (normal)	At 37 weeks (abnormal)
Light reflexes	Absent	Absent
Respirations	Periodic breathing	Periodic breathing
Muscle tone	Low in extremities	Low in extremities
Evaluation	Normal for age	CNS stress

TABLE 7. Differentiating between Jitteriness and
Seizures in the Newborn

Finding	Jitteriness	Seizures
Deviation of eyes	No	Yes
Reaction to stimuli	Yes	No
Movements rhythmic	Yes	No
Controlled by holding	Yes	No

TABLE 8. The First 72 hr after the Asphyxia–Ischemic Stress

Time	Respirations	Muscle tone	Eyes	Seizures	Sensorium
<12 hr	Apneic spells Cheyne-Stokes	Hypotonia	Fixed, blinking	Present after 6–12 hr in 50% of cases	Depressed
>12 hr	Periodic	Low tone Hypotonia	Intact pupillary response	Present	Stupor to coma
12–24 hr	Apneic spells	Jittery (controlled by holding)	Fixed	Present tonic or tonic–clonic Myoclonic	Stuporous
24–72 hr	Respiratory arrest Apnea	Flaccid	Loss of eye response to doll's head maneuver	Present	Remains stuporous
After 72 hr	Irregular, periodic	Disturbed sucking and gag reflexes	Oculomotor changes	Less frequent	Less stuporous in survivals to deep coma in brain dead
Prognosis	Brain death, cerebral palsy, IVH in prematures Hydrocephalus				

STAGE I

Mild hypoxia (low P_{O_2})
Low O_2 supply
Mild asphyxia
No CNS symptoms

STAGE II

Moderate asphyxia
Hypoxia (low P_{O_2})
CO_2 retention
Hypercapnia (high P_{O_2})

Moderate CNS involvement
   Low tone
   Depression of
      cardiorespiratory centers

STAGE III

Hypoxia (low P_{O_2})
Hypercapnia (high P_{CO_2})
Metabolic acidosis

Serious CNS involvement
   Depression
   Coma
   Seizures
   Brain death

FIGURE 2. Crucial stages of central nervous system asphyxia.

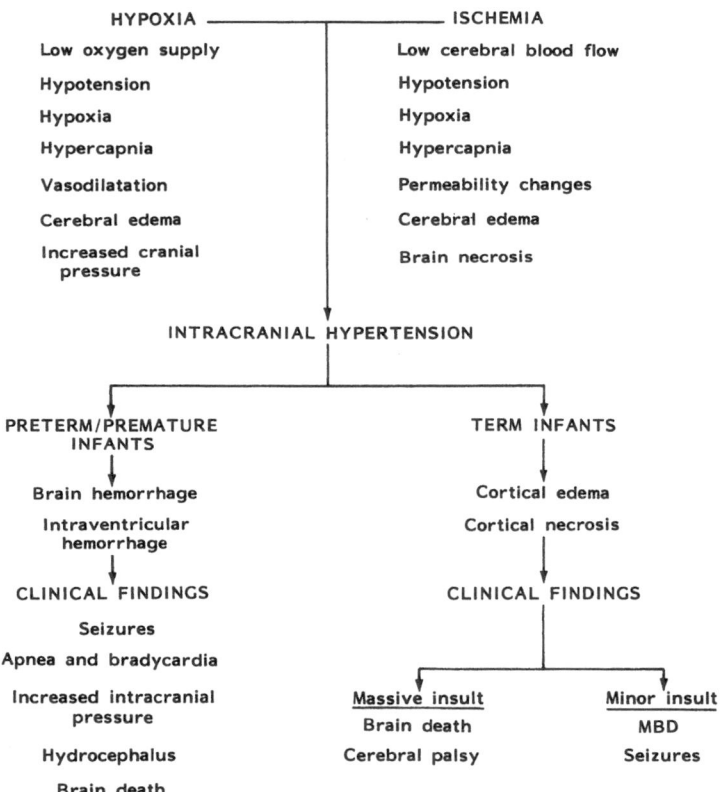

FIGURE 3. Effects of hypoxia and asphyxia on the CNS.

this baby does not develop twitching, then the prognosis would be a good future or minor neurological deficits as he develops, either delayed milestones or MBD behavior. The Apgar score in this stage would be 5.

Stage 3 Asphyxia

This is a baby born with severe compromise at birth, flaccid, cyanotic, and apneic at birth, not responding to stimuli, and with severe bradycardia. This baby represents an example of severe birth asphyxia with its expression involving major systems: CNS (neurological), respiratory, metabolic, and cardiovascular. The prognosis for this baby is very serious, and mortality is about 50%.

If the baby recovers from this crucial period through a well-planned course of therapy, he may survive, but his prognosis is guarded and can only be defined as he develops.

The degree of damage can only be determined by tests (CSF, CAT scan, neurological work-up, sonography) and will also depend on the degree of maturity: prognosis is more reserved in premature infants under 32 weeks of gestation and with birth weights under 1200 g, who are very susceptible to brain hemorrhage. In this group of asphyxiated newborns, the prognosis is for survival, but complications of asphyxia are many, and such sequelae of bleeding as hydrocephalus are a real possibility.

Brain Hemorrhage

If brain hemorrhage occurs before 26 weeks of gestation, its major effect is on the white matter; within the range of 24 to 31 weeks of gestation, brain hemorrhage affects the germinal matrix. In a term infant, brain hemorrhage may manifest as a subarachnoid hemorrhage.

In prematures less than 1200 g at birth, brain hemorrhages can be classified according to extent: type I affects the germinal layer; type II is intraventricular (IVH); type III includes IVH plus hydrocephalus; type IV affects the parenchyma in addition to producing IVH and hydrocephalus. This classification correlates with the clinical symptoms. Type I brain hemorrhage may produce no symptoms or only mild neurological abnormalities. Type II may produce no symptoms or, in up to 50% of cases, mild neurological symptoms including apneas, bradycardias, and jitteriness. Types III and IV can produce hearing deficits, blindness, hydrocephalus, seizures (tonic, multifocal, clonic, or myoclonic), and CP.

Effects of Asphyxia on the Brain in the Newborn Period

The brain can be deficient in oxygen because of hypoxemia (lack of oxygen in the blood) or ischemia (lack of blood supply).

Effects of Hypoxemia on the Brain

1. Increased vascular permeability.
2. Vascular dilatation, swelling, and edema of the brain tissue, which can be responsible for inadequate blood supply.
3. Increased glucose uptake and lactic acid production.

4. Greater effects on the brainstem and hypothalamus, which are more sensitive to hypoxic insult than the cerebral cortex.
5. Alterations in the mechanism of thermoregulation and respiratory regulation (and change in color of the newborn) as a result of effects on hypothalamus and brainstem.

Effects of Ischemia on the Brain

1. Depletion of glucose stores.
2. Lactic acid accumulation and acidosis.
3. Vasodilatation does *not* occur.
4. Cerebral damage possibly leading to brain death if perfusion is not improved.
5. Postrecovery sequelae of the ischemic stress:
   a. Spastic paresis.
   b. Visual or auditory defects.
   c. Seizures.
   d. Psychomotor retardation of varying degrees.

7

Brain Asphyxia and Hemorrhage

The fetus is oxygenated by a system of mixed blood. Oxygen supply depends on the oxygen that is transported by the umbilical vein (UV), which originates at the level of the intervillous space of the placenta, where oxygen and CO_2 are exchanged.

The UV carries highly oxygenated blood to the liver. There, oxygenated blood from the UV shunts at the level of the ductus venosus (DV) with the inferior vena cava (IVC), and the liver gets well-oxygenated blood. Shunting at the DV and IVC creates mixed blood. The IVC shunts with the superior vena cava (SVC), which drains nonoxygenated blood from the brain and upper extremities; both drain into the right atrium (RA). At the level of the RA blood shunts via the foramen ovale (FO) to the left atrium (LA), left ventricle (LV), and aorta. Venous pressure higher than systemic pressure creates a right-to-left shunt in fetal life.

The heart receives less oxygenated blood than the liver. From the RA to RV and via the pulmonary artery (PA), the blood shunts to the aorta via the patent ductus

arteriosus (PDA). Less-oxygenated blood shunts via the
FO and PDA and is distributed from the aorta to the
brain and all body tissues. Thus, the best-oxygenated organs are the liver, heart, and brain, more than the tissues of the gastrointestinal tract, lungs, and limbs.

Asphyxial stress owing to systemic maternal causes,
obstetric causes, or placental or umbilical cord compression, particularly during delivery, creates increased pulmonary vascular resistance, which establishes the right-
to-left shunt characteristic of persistent fetal circulation
(PFC) in the hypoxic fetus.

In asphyxial–ischemic stress, different types of
pathology occur in very-low-birth-weight (VLBW) infants
than in those that are full term. Damage created by
hypoxic ischemic stress in the central nervous system
will depend on the duration of the stress and the age of
the fetus.

Asphyxia and Ischemia

Asphyxia and ischemia as causes of central nervous
system (CNS) lesions differ in VLBW and in full-term infants. In VLBW infants the lesions occur intraventricu-
larly and in the gray nuclei, caudate nuclei, thalamus,
germinal matrix, and lateral and third ventricles. In full-
term infants, lesions are observed in the gray matter
(necrosis), cerebrum, and cerebellum.

Hypoxia

Severe hypoxia in the first trimester of gestation may
cause embryonic or fetal death. It may produce malfor-

mations as a result of tissue hypoxia that may be responsible for brain necrosis and different degrees of anomalies in the developing brain.

In VLBW, anoxia causing brain hemorrhage predominantly affects the matrix zone, which is located between the caudate nucleus and the thalamus, at the level of the foramina of Monro. It connects the lateral ventricles with the third ventricle. Sometimes, brain hemorrhage affecting the matrix zone extends to the medial aspects of the lateral ventricles, which are extensions of the matrix zone.

Veins originating in this area are very fragile and resemble capillaries with poor stroma. Neurons and glia of the cerebral cortex and basal ganglia originate in the germinal matrix.

In summary, brain hemorrhage in the VLBW infant is favored by hypoxia and hypercarbia secondary to hyaline membrane disease (HMD), requiring mechanical respirators.

Clinical Aspects of Brain Hemorrhage

The diagnosis of brain hemorrhage affecting VLBW infants may be entertained when the following clinical findings are present:

1. Cardiovascular:
   a. Sudden pallor.
   b. Hypotension.
   c. Bradycardia.
   d. Apneas with bradycardia (A&B).
2. Neurological:
   a. Marked hypotonia.

   b. Sudden paresis or quadriparesis.
   c. Coma.
   d. Decerebrate posture.
   e. Seizures.
   f. Fixed pupils.
   g. Signs of intracranial hypertension.
3. Intracranial hemorrhage as documented by work-up:
   a. Head sonogram.
   b. CAT scan.
   c. CSF (spinal tap): ↑XHb, ↑XRBCs.
   d. EEG showing spikes in the Roland region as an expression of brain hemorrhage affecting the matrix zone.
4. Hematologic: ↓XHb, ↓XHct.
5. Respiratory: ↓XpH, ↑XCO$_2$, ↓XPO$_2$; respiratory acidosis.
6. Metabolic: ↓XpH, ↓XHCO$_3$, ↓XPO$_2$; metabolic acidosis.
7. Calcium: low.
8. Renal: low output, elevated BUN and creatinine, which may represent hypoperfusion, shock, or metabolic acidosis; may cause renal failure if prolonged.

Brain Hemorrhage in the Newborn

Clinical signs of brain hemorrhage in the newborn depend on the location of the hemorrhage. Intraventricular hemorrhage (IVH) can cause coma, decerebrate posturing, tonic seizures, apnea, fixed pupils, paralysis, and risk of hydrocephalus. Periventricular leukomalacia may cause lower limb weakness. Parasagittal cerebral necrosis may lead to hip and shoulder weakness. Lesions of the cerebellum, thalamus, and brainstem nuclei may cause stupor, coma, and disturbed sucking reflexes.

Histopathology of the Brain under Anoxia

Histopathological lesions can result from traumatic delivery. Trauma to shoulders and abdomen can lead to congestion and leptomeninges. Head trauma can cause subdural hemorrhage. Birth anoxia can cause subarachnoid hemorrhage. Anoxia in the premature causes lesions of the hippocampus, dentate and amygdaloid nuclei, and Purkinje layer of the cerebellum.

Anoxia and hypoxia in the more mature premature infant can affect white matter and nerve cells. Lesions may be seen over the periventricular frontotemporo-occipital areas described as "foci of leukomalacia"; these are found in 40% of premature infants suffering from HMD or RDS. Postgliosis follows this stage; it is recognized as poorly myelinated areas near ventricles. Anoxia and hypoxia can also produce brain hemorrhage in these infants.

Asphyxia in the premature is also a cause of hemorrhage affecting the lateral ventricles. Immature neuroblastic and glial tissues give little support to the great vein of Galen, which is an area where hemorrhage is often seen. In severe hemorrhage, blood may drain into ventricles and the subarachnoid space and then from the third and fourth ventricles into the medulla. In the VLBW group (<1200 g) with a history of HMD or RDS, the possibility of brain hemorrhage must be considered if jitteriness, apnea, or convulsions appear after 24 hr of respiratory distress.

Fetal Muscle Tone *in Utero* and in the Newborn

During gestation, the appearance of flexor muscle tone progresses in the cephalad direction. At 25–26 weeks of gestation, flexor tone appears in the legs, at 30 weeks in the thighs (legs are flexed), and at 34 weeks in the upper limbs (all four extremities are flexed). At 36 weeks, the flexor tone of the extremities is increased, and at 38 weeks, thigh adduction becomes apparent. By 40 weeks, flexor tone is predominant in the limbs.

Muscle tone in the newborn is a reflection of CNS health or insult (asphyxia, trauma, infection, metabolic factors, or sedation or anesthesia in the mother). Hypotonia in the newborn reflects hypoxia or mild asphyxia. Spasticity at birth implies longstanding hypoxic insult (e.g., prolonged intrauterine infection). Low tone followed by spasticity indicates a course of CNS asphyxia over a few weeks. Low tone with areflexia and depression indicates severe asphyxia, sedation, or a metabolic cause; however, low tone and areflexia in an alert newborn imply myopathy or anterior horn disease. Low muscle tone with dysmorphic features signifies a genetic or chromosomal dysfunction (e.g., trisomy 21). Low tone with A&B in a VLBW newborn indicates asphyxia and/or brain hemorrhage.

8

Types and Stages of Fetal Anoxia
Anoxic, Anemic, Stagnant, and Histotoxic

Anoxia means lack of adequate oxygenation. There are four types of anoxia (Figs. 4 and 5) that may interfere with the mechanism of oxygenation and cause inadequate ventilation of the fetus.

Anoxic Anoxia

Anoxic anoxia represents a problem of inadequate oxygenation of the fetus as a result of systemic causes in the mother. These include problems related to ventilatory mechanisms in the mother such as respiratory and/or cardiovascular conditions, hypertension, or toxemia. Anoxic anoxia also arises from obstetric causes such as placental factors that may interfere with oxygen transport at the level of the umbilical cord, cord compression or mechanical factors such as cord around the neck

ANOXIC ANOXIA

Poor oxygen supply
or exchange,
hypoventilation

ANEMIC ANOXIA

Inadequate oxygenation
because of insufficient
amount of RBC or Hb
to carry oxygen

STAGNANT ANOXIA

Inadequate oxygenation
because blood does not
circulate fast enough
in blood vessels because
of heart failure

HISTOTOXIC ANOXIA

Oxygen supply is
sufficient but not
utilized by tissues
because of cell toxicity

FIGURE 4. Types of anoxia.

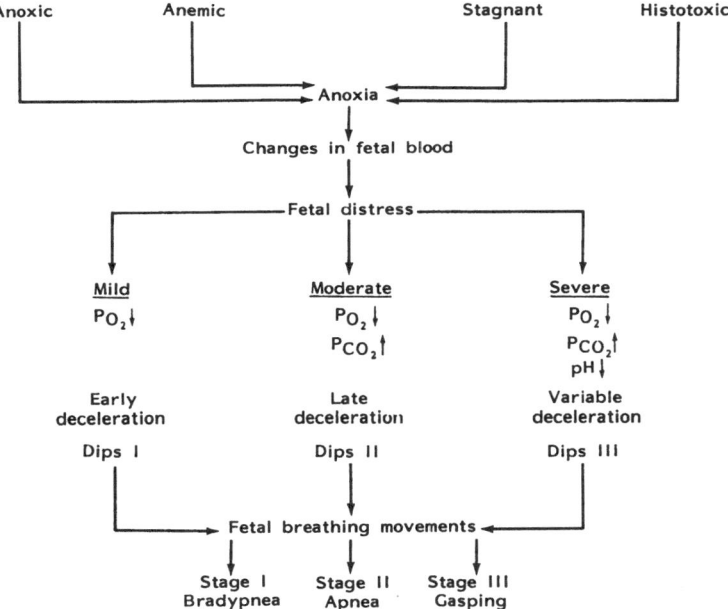

FIGURE 5. Stages of fetal anoxia and their relationship to observations by fetal monitoring.

that compromise adequate oxygenation because of the blocking of the umbilical cord, cord prolapse, uterine dysfunction, failure of the uterine muscles to contract, cephalopelvic disproportion, or any anomaly of presentation during the time of delivery.

In these cases, there is also inadequate blood oxygenation, and therefore the fetus is compromised by poor oxygen flow.

Anemic Anoxia

In anemic anoxia there is an adequate amount of oxygen; the oxygen is available, but the transport of this oxygen is insufficient. This could arise from a deficit in hemoglobin and/or an inadequate number of red blood cells (anemias).

The causes of anemic anoxia include bleeding diathesis, systemic bleeding of the mother, obstetric bleeding such as from placenta previa, an abruptio placenta, which represents a separation of the placenta before the baby is born, and/or a trauma, either systemic or obstetric.

In these examples, anoxia is related to a significant anemia, but there are also cases of anemic anoxia related to hemolysis. Factors that cause hemolysis—hemoglobinopathies, erythroblastosis fetalis, thalassemia, or sickle cell crisis—create a significant reduction in the total amount of hemoglobin and therefore a significant risk to oxygen transport. In other words, any factor that leads to a deficit in the number of red blood cells or amount of hemoglobin or both can cause anemic anoxia.

Stagnant Anoxia

There is a third type of anoxia that arises from a cardiovascular mechanism. The blood does not move in the vessels fast enough to guarantee adequate O_2 transfer. The cause of this type of anoxia is cardiac failure causing poor perfusion and therefore not allowing the blood to circulate with the frequency and volume required. This will cause a deficit of oxygen secondary to insufficient blood supply, which is called stagnant anoxia.

Histotoxic Anoxia

Here, the lack of oxygenation is caused by lack of utilization of oxygen by the cells even though the blood and oxygen supply is adequate. In this type of anoxia, tissues do not absorb the oxygen offered because of cell or tissue poisoning. An example is barbiturate poisoning; the utilization of oxygen is blocked by pharmacological tissue toxicity.

Fetal Decelerations

Any of these types of anoxia—anoxic, anemic, stagnant, and histotoxic—or possible combinations of them decompensate and create circulatory collapse. An example of anoxic anoxia *in utero* is the case of anoxia affecting a fetus during labor owing to obstetric causes; the fetus becomes hypoxic because of the prolonged labor and dystocias of labor. During prolonged contractions, there is insufficient blood flow through the placenta and umbilical cord; the problem can be detected by cardiac monitoring. This is what Caldeyro-Barcia calls fetal decelerations, and he divides these into three types.

Type I: Early Deceleration

At the peak of uterine contractions, the pulse slows. If the hypoxia is progressive, we have type II deceleration.

Type II: Late Deceleration

The fetal pulse slows to bradycardia, which continues after the uterine contraction is over. This represents a more severe type of hypoxia or a more prolonged asphyxial stress. In this case, there are hypoxia (lack of oxygen) and CO_2 retention (hypercapnia). If the asphyxial stress is still more prolonged, it produces the third type of asphyxia, ''variable deceleration.''

Type III: Variable Decelerations

The fetal heart rate is low for a longer time (Caldeyro-Barcia's Dips III), which represents prolonged fetal asphyxia with hypoxia, hypercapnia, and metabolic acidosis.

Summary

In mild fetal anoxia (early deceleration, Dips I), deceleration occurs at the peak of uterine contractions. In persistent anoxia (late fetal deceleration, Dips II), the deceleration is prolonged after the contraction, and there is low O_2 and CO_2 retention. In serious anoxia (variable deceleration, Dips III), the fetal pulse is slow, under 100 beats/min, for a prolonged period, and there is a lack of O_2 and retention of CO_2 (hypercapnia and metabolic acidosis).

By the use of ultrasound, it has been documented (A-scan technique) that there are fetal breathing movements (FBM) *in utero*. If the fetus is receiving an adequate oxygen supply, fetal breathing movements are regular. This has been recorded clearly in multigravida in the last weeks of pregnancy and in adequate-for-gestational-age (AGA) babies. If the fetus is under fetal distress because of hypoxia, then the baby's FBM become irregular to parallel fetal deceleration in monitoring.

Finally, if the hypoxia persists, there is a gasping pattern; the fetus may die *in utero* unless delivered immediately. This stage of gasping corresponds to deceleration type III or variable deceleration. Arterial blood gas monitoring shows low pH, low PO_2, high PCO_2, and low HCO_3^-, representing combined respiratory and metabolic acidosis, an expression of severe asphyxia.

9

Embryonic and Fetal Periods

The embryonic period, extending from conception to the ninth week of gestation, is an active period of growth and formation of different organs and systems. Inadequate blood flow or oxygen deprivation during this period of time may have significant effects on embryo formation (Figs. 6–9).

Fertilization and Stages of Embryo Development

From the moment the egg (oocyte) is fertilized by the spermatozoa, it changes into a new form, called a zygote. This takes place at the level of the Fallopian tubes. From this moment a period of active cellular division and growth of the zygote begins.

In the process of descending from the Fallopian tubes to the uterine cavity for its implantation, the zygote moves slowly. This journey is facilitated by peristaltic movements of the fimbria of the tubal walls.

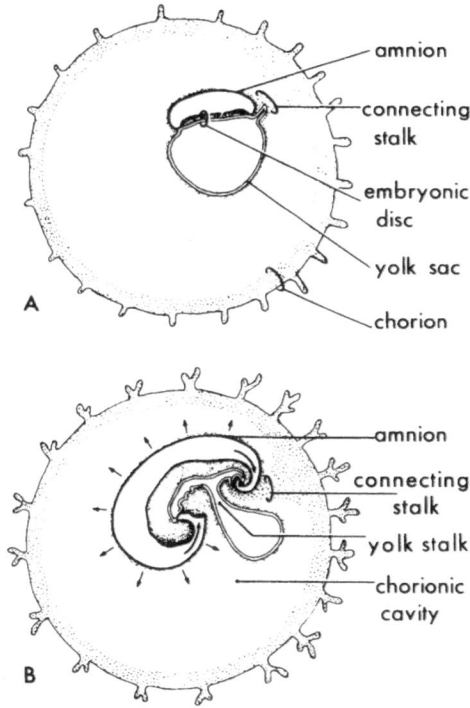

FIGURE 6. Growth of fetal membranes. A and B show expansion of the amnion covering the embryo, yolk sac, and umbilical cord. C and D show progressive growth of the amniotic cavity covering the umbili-

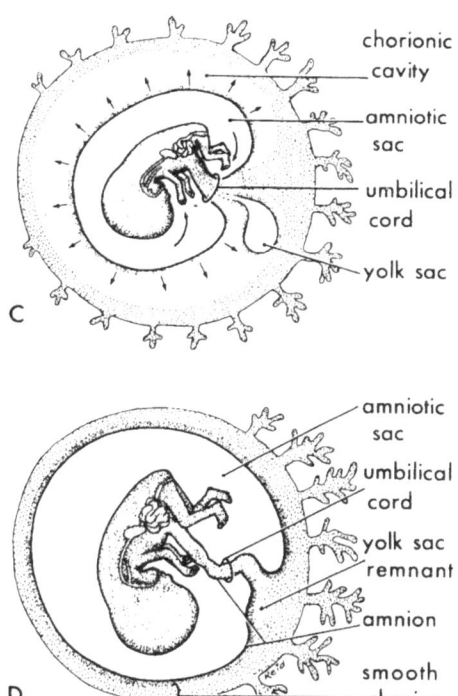

cal cord and show how the yolk sac is incorporated as the primitive intestine. (From Moore, 1977, p. 127, with permission.)

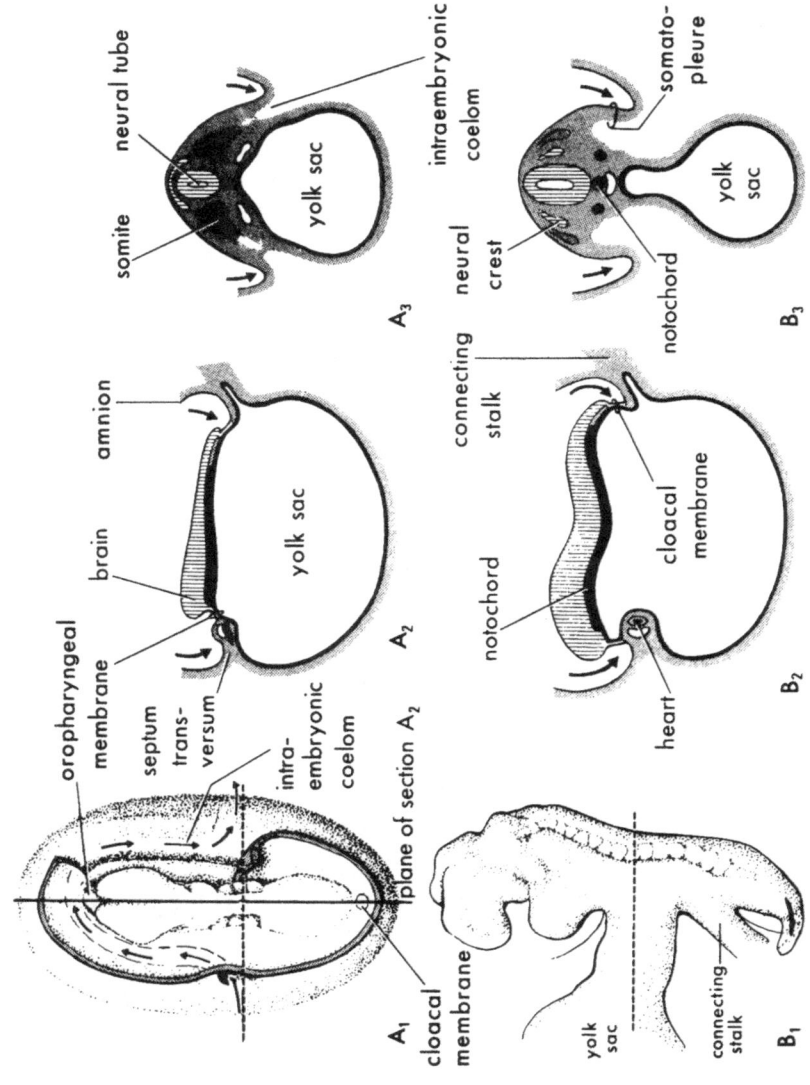

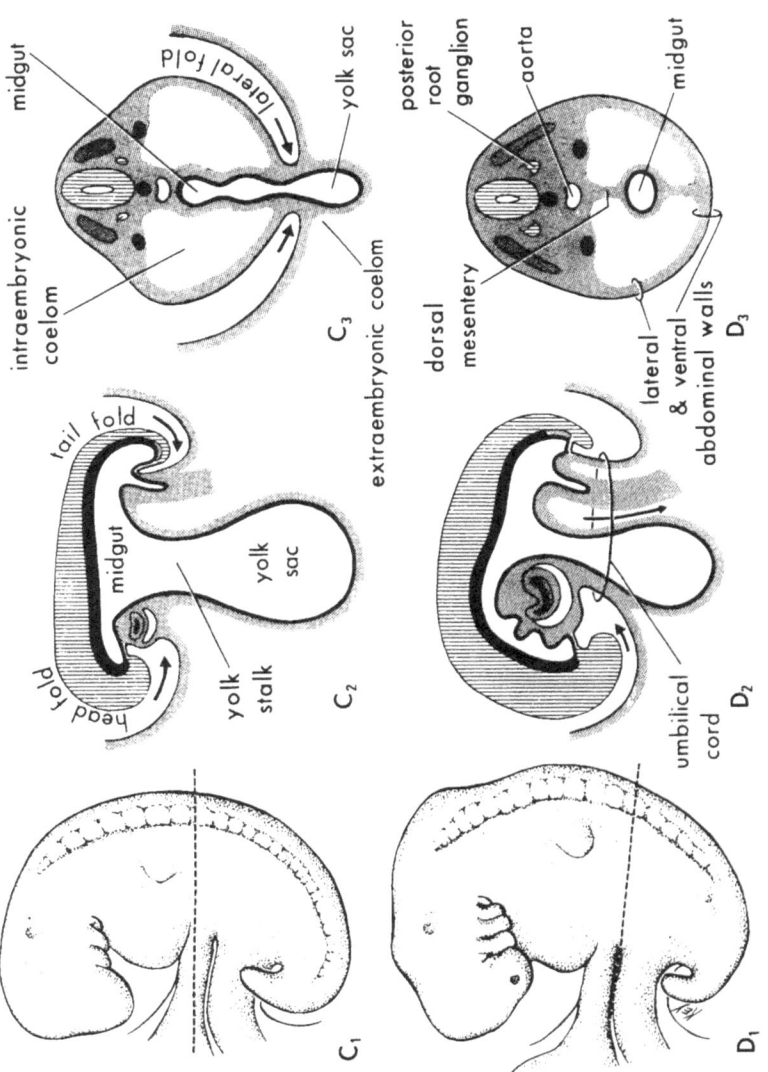

FIGURE 7. Period of embryonic development of central nervous system, heart, and digestive system: fourth week. (From Moore, 1977, p. 71, with permission.)

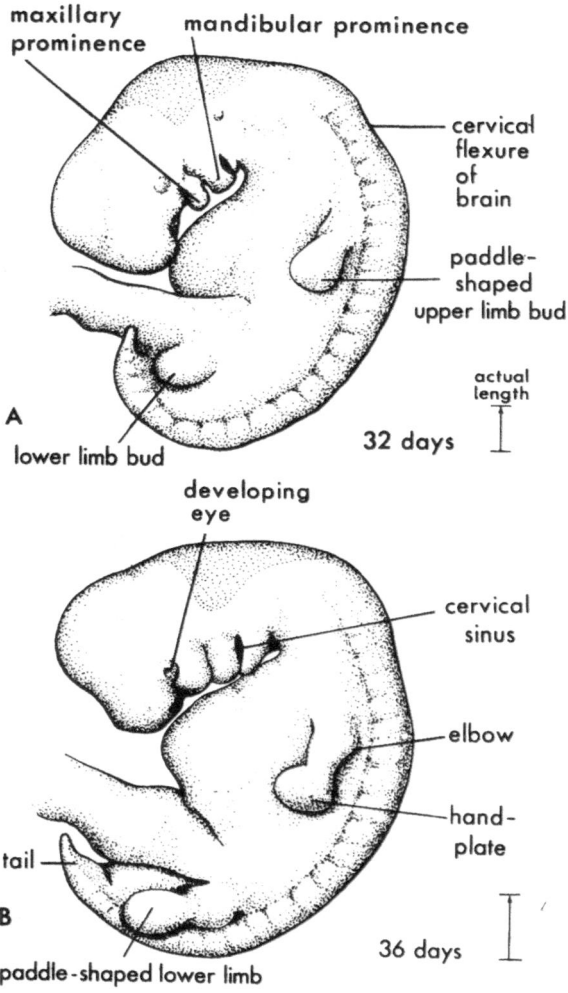

maxillary prominence

mandibular prominence

cervical flexure of brain

paddle-shaped upper limb bud

actual length

A

lower limb bud

32 days

developing eye

cervical sinus

elbow

hand-plate

tail

B

36 days

paddle-shaped lower limb

FIGURE 8. Embryonic development of sensory organs and extremities: weeks 4 to 8. (From Moore, 1977, p. 84, with permission.)

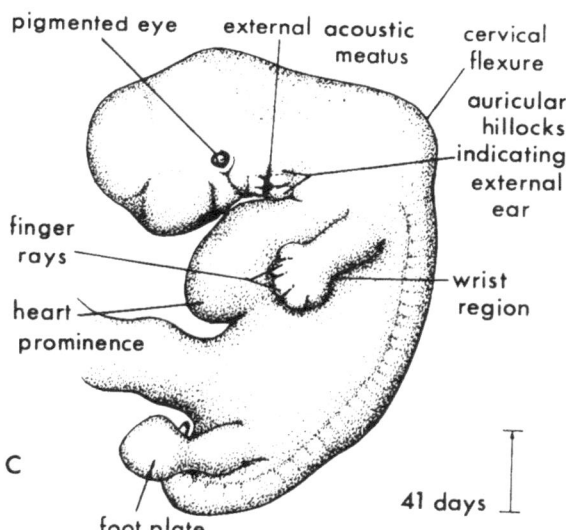

FIGURE 8. (*continued*)

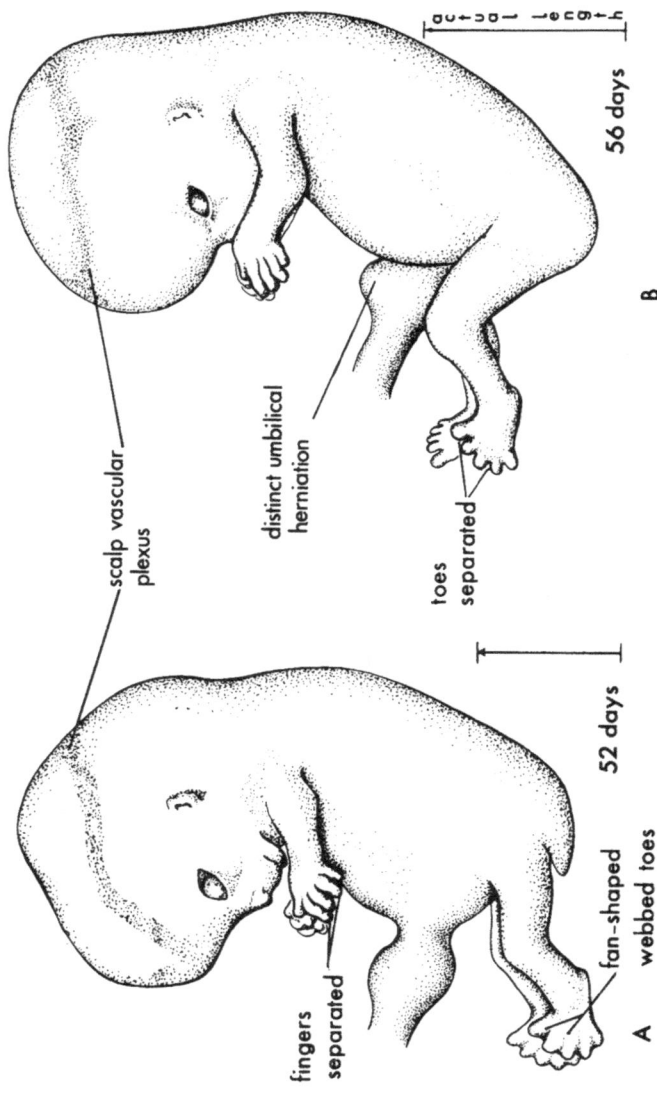

FIGURE 9. End of embryonic period: formation of fingers and toes. (From Moore, 1977, p. 88, with permission.)

An active process of cell division takes place. From two cells that constitute the zygote (egg and spermatozoa), the cells will divide into 4, 8, 12, 24. At this stage the zygote is called a morula, from the Latin for mulberry. By this time the fertilized zygote is 5 or 6 days old and reaches the uterine mucosa (inner part of the uterine wall) for its nidation or implantation.

As cell division proceeds, there is a realignment of cells forming a hollow-ball-like cell grouping, called a blastocyst. The layer of cells that will be in contact with the uterine wall is the trophoblast, which will form the placenta. The group of inner cells of the blastocyst will form the embryoblast and the fetus. Therefore, both fetus and placenta will originate from the primitive zygote.

From the moment of nidation or implantation in the uterine mucosa (day 6 or 7), the trophoblast will start to dig deeply into the uterine wall, trying to establish a vascular connection between the mother's circulation and the growing embryo. At this time the original trophoblast divides into two types of cells: syncytiotrophoblasts, high columnar types of cells that try to establish a deep connection with the vessels of the uterine mucosa, and cuboidal types of cells called cytotrophoblasts, the inner layer of cells which will form the endoderm. At the same time, other types of cells originating in the trophoblast will form the chorion, which will be the external wall that will separate the embryo from the uterine mucosa.

The union of the cytotrophoblast and the sincytiotrophoblast will form the embryonic disk. By then, the embryo is 12–13 days old.

As the connection between the syncyciotrophoblast and the uterus deepens, this area will form the future placenta. Also, a vascular connection called the body stalk will be established and will eventually become the umbilical cord.

Close to the third week of age (18th to 19th day), the embryonic disk grows in length and develops a pear shape. A fissure at the level of the ectoderm layer is formed. This layer of cells extends laterally and will give origin to the mesoderm. By then, the embryo is 3 weeks old.

At 3 weeks of age the embryo is about 1/8 inch long. By this time three layers of cells are formed:

1. Ectoderm, which originates from the syncytiotrophoblasts.
2. Endoderm, which originates from the cytotrophoblasts.
3. Mesoderm, the layer that will be established between the ectoderm and the endoderm.

From the syncytiotrophoblast or external layer, the amnion and the amniotic cavity will also develop; these will cover the embryo as the inner expanding cavity that will gradually occupy the space of the original chorionic cavity.

From the ectoderm are derived skin, hair, nails, central nervous system, the sensory organs, the mouth, and the anus.

From the mesoderm are derived muscle, bone, upper urinary tract, reproductive system, cardiovascular system, and blood-forming organs of the hematopoietic system.

From the endoderm originate the gastrointestinal system, the tonsils, thymus, thyroid gland, parathyroid glands, and lower urinary tract.

At 27–30 days of age, the embryo begins to show rapid head growth; the heart starts to beat; the limb buds and legs appear. The umbilical cord is already present. The amniotic cavity starts to grow and will gradually replace the space originally occupied by the chorionic cavity.

At 6 weeks, the embryo is 5 mm long. At 8 weeks, the embryo is 1 cm long. At 9 weeks, the embryo length is 5 cm. This marks the end of the embryo period or the ninth week of gestation, with the completion of the head, eyes, heart, and the formation of the extremities.

Teratogenic Factors

Teratogenic factors are aggressive factors for the vitality of the embryo and fetus undergoing formation. They include physical factors, chemical factors, and infectious and nutritional factors. These different etiologies may create changes in such forming systems and organs as CNS, sensory organs, heart, limbs, and genitalia.

There are many mechanisms of action, but interference in nutrition and oxygenation is crucial, particularly in the embryonic stage more than in the fetal period, because by then the major organs and systems are already formed.

10

The Placenta
Origin and Functions

Because of the many roles of the placenta (nutrition, en-docrine, renal), it is without question a key organ in the process of fetal oxygenation. Its performance may be the key to fetal well-being and good growth, or a deficit in fetal nutrition with asphyxial stress (see Fig. 10).

Formation and Functions of the Placenta

The placenta originates in the trophoblast group of cells that we have already described in the original zy-gote, which was the fertilized ovum. After fertilization, cell division creates the morula stage.

In the blastocyst stage, the trophoblast represents the original wall of the blastocyst, which will then, through the process of nidation, be surrounded by the uterine

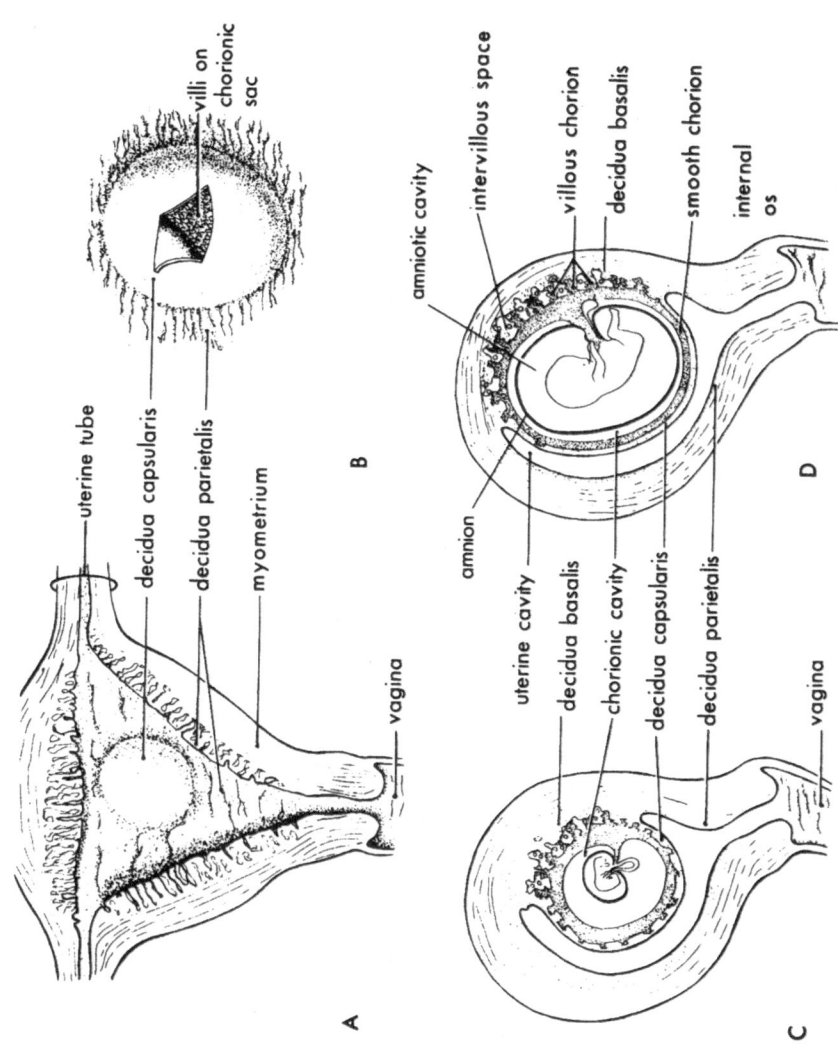

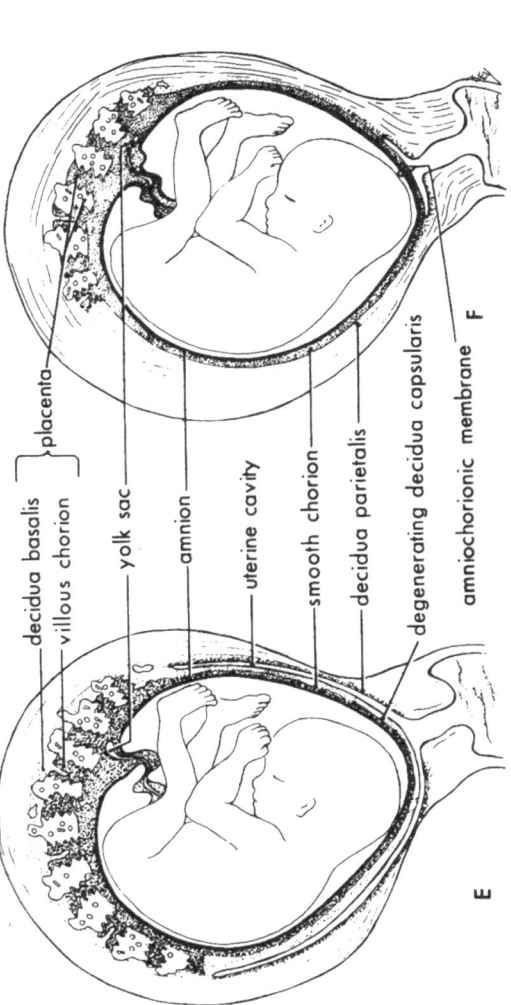

FIGURE 10. Fetal membrane and placenta. In the uterine mucosa, after nidation of the fertilized oocyte, the blastocyst originates the decidua basalis, the future placenta. The decidua capsularis is the membrane that covers the amnion and chorion, which are the membranes that immediately surround the fetus. (From Moore, 1977, p. 121, with permission.)

mucosa. By a process of proteolysis, the zygote will then finally be implanted in the uterine mucosa.

From the trophoblast will originate the decidua basalis, which in turn is the origin of the placenta. The placenta thus has a fetal origin. It is nothing but a process of thickening of the original trophoblast.

From its formation in the third week of gestation, the function of the placenta is well established.

At this level arterial and venous capillaries establish communication between the mother and the fetus, and through the placenta, a vital process of interchange of oxygen and nutrients will take place that will allow the embryo and later on the fetus to grow to become the future baby at birth.

The placenta plays a major role in the process of fetal oxygenation. The lungs do not perform any oxygen interchange during fetal life. Instead, exchanges of oxygen occur through the villi of the placenta.

The umbilical vein carries oxygen from the placenta to the fetus, and umbilical arteries return the carbon dioxide for gas exchange at the level of the placenta. Therefore, the placenta is equivalent to the fetal lungs in the important role of oxygenation throughout fetal life.

Another role of the placenta is its nutritional function. The placenta provides to the fetus such elements as amino acids, fatty acids, phospholipids, and lipoproteins—all essential in filling the nutritional requirements of the embryo and the fetus for total growth.

A third role of the placenta is that of renal function. The fetus produces urine from the fourth month of gestation; 500 ml of urine is filtered per day in the ninth month of gestation. This urine that the fetus produces drains into the amniotic fluid; the fetus swallows this and it is reabsorbed by the intestine, and returns to the placenta via the umbilical arteries for exchange with the maternal circulation.

A fourth role of the placenta is an endocrine or glandular one. The placenta produces a hormone called chorionic gonadotropin, whose function is to guarantee the nidation of the zygote of the fertilized ovum in the uterus. This function is in a way similar to that of the corpus luteum of the ovary. Chorionic gonadotropin production is documented from the sixth day postnidation of the zygote in the uterine mucosa. Peak production occurs in the second month of pregnancy, and it declines after the fifth month. The presence of this substance in the blood and urine of the mother shortly after a missed menstrual period is a valid test for early confirmation of pregnancy.

Other endocrine functions of the placenta include the production of progesterone. Progesterone of placental origin gives vitality to the endometrium and will guarantee the normal process of gestation. The placenta also produces estrogens. Since these estrogens are maternal–fetal in origin, their presence will indirectly reflect the well-being and good growth of the fetus. Lower levels of placental estrogens and lower levels of estriol in the blood and urine of the mother are an indication of stress or difficulties or, indirectly, lack of fetal well-being.

The placenta at term has a length of 15–20 cm, a thickness of 2–3 cm, and a weight of 400–500 g. The inner part of the placenta is called the amnion. The external side is called the chorion. The chorionic villi are observed in the external part of the placenta, which is the portion of the placenta that is in contact with the uterine mucosa. The inner part of the placenta, the amnion, produces the amniotic fluid that covers the fetus.

The umbilical cord develops from the chorionic villi, which grow in size from small capillary elements to become the two umbilical arteries and the one umbilical vein.

The umbilical cord has a length of 50–55 cm and a width of about 2–3 cm (20 inches long by a width of 1 inch). The umbilical cord is formed by the one umbilical vein that carries oxygenated blood from the placenta to the fetus and by the umbilical arteries that return nonoxygenated or venous blood from the fetus to the placenta. The two umbilical arteries and the umbilical vein are surrounded by a jellylike substance called Wharton's jelly, which protects the vessels from trauma. The elastic fibers of the arterial wall will aid the hemostatic mechanism by constriction when the umbilical cord is clamped and cut.

The flow of blood in the umbilical cord is about 200–300 ml/min at the end of pregnancy. There is no pain sensitivity at the level of the umbilical cord. There are no actual nerve endings, which explains the absence of pain when the cord is clamped and cut.

Mechanisms of Maternal–Fetal Exchange through the Placenta

The placenta is the bridge between the maternal and fetal circulations. Oxygenated blood from the mother reaches the fetus through the uterine arterioles and is exchanged via the placenta to the umbilical vein, which carries oxygen to the fetus (see Table 9). Deoxygenated blood from the fetus is exchanged at the level of the intervillous space of the placenta and is returned to the placenta from the two umbilical arteries.

Maternal uterine arterioles spread through the intervillous space. Maternal and fetal blood do not mix, for there is a thin membrane that separates them. The intervillous space is the area where the exchange of oxygen and carbon dioxide takes place and nutrients are provided to the fetus. At the same time, in this area, renal wastes coming along the umbilical arteries from the fetus are exchanged. Therefore, the intervillous space is the liaison area and the exchange zone.

These then are the four roles of the placenta:

1. Oxygenation, giving oxygenated blood to the fetus.
2. Nutrition, giving nutrients to the fetus.
3. Renal function at the level of the intervillous space, where fetal renal wastes are exchanged and elimination of waste products takes place.
4. Endocrine or glandular function.

The Placenta during Labor

It has been well documented that during uterine contractions in labor, blood perfusion diminishes at the intervillous space, as do oxygenation and the blood oxygen tension. This stage of uterine contractions causes a fetal deceleration that is parallel to the degree and duration of contraction. This is a crucial period for the fetus.

TABLE 9. Mechanism of Fetal Oxygenation and Nutrition during Pregnancy and Delivery

Mother	Placenta bridge/intervillous space	Fetus
During pregnancy		
Maternal uterine arterioles	↑→→→→→→→→→→→→→→→→→→→→→→↑↑↑↑↑	Umbilical vein receives oxygen and nutrients and carries them to fetus
Placental roles		
• Oxygenation	→→→→→→→→	Exchange zone for oxygen and nutrients →→
• Nutrition		
• Renal		
Uterine vein ←←←←←←←←←←←←←←←←←←←	CO_2 ←←←←←←←←←←←←←←←←←←←← Renal function	Two umbilical arteries carry nonoxygenated, CO_2-rich blood to the placenta; clearance of renal wastes

In normal delivery

Uterine contraction	→→→→→→ ↑↑	Blood is injected through the intervillous space	Causes fetal deceleration
Uterine artery	→→→→→→→→→→→→→→→→→→		Oxygen is received by umbilical vein
Nonoxygenated blood is received by uterine vein	↓↓↓↓↓↓↓↓↓↓↓↓↓↓↓↓↓↓↓↓		Umbilical arteries deliver nonoxygenated, CO_2-rich blood to the placenta

If abnormal uterine contractions occur

Placental insufficiency	→→→→→→→→→→ ↑	Oxygen and CO_2 exchange is impaired at the intervillous space	Causes fetal asphyxia
Poor oxygen saturation[a]	→→→→→→→→→→→→→→→→→→→→→		Causes CO_2 accumulation

[a]Maternal factors that may cause poor oxygenation at delivery include cardiovascular disease, respiratory disease, severe anemia, and impaired renal function.

Oxygen exchange and level of CO_2 (nonoxygenated blood) will depend on (1) blood flow at the intervillous space, (2) diffusion capacity of the placenta and area of exchange, and (3) oxygen tension of uterine artery and umbilical vessels. Anomalies in placental anatomy such as small size of the placenta, fibrosis of the placenta, and a placenta with areas of calcification may affect placental functions and may interfere with performance in this particular stage. Therefore, there is a risk in oxygenating the fetus well and in exchanging CO_2. The end result is asphyxia and metabolic acidosis of the fetus at birth.

In addition to the factors interfering in good exchange that are related directly to placental size and function, there are general factors that may create deficits in oxygenating the fetus:

1. Cardiovascular disease of the mother.
2. Respiratory disease of the mother, causing poor ventilation.
3. Poor maternal renal function.
4. Severe anemias of the mother.

In all these cases the oxygen content (arterial oxygen) of the mother is diminished, and therefore oxygen exchange at the level of the placenta will be reduced, causing fetal asphyxia.

11

Fetal Circulation

Oxygenated blood from the placenta in the umbilical vein shunts at the level of the liver through the ductus venosus and from there flows into the inferior vena cava (IVC). The IVC and the superior vena cava (SVC) both drain into the right atrium (RA). From the right atrium, the oxygenated blood goes via the tricuspid valve to the right ventricle, and from there it enters the pulmonary artery. A small portion goes to the lungs, not for exchange but to supply oxygen and blood to the lungs.

Because of the high pulmonary vascular resistance that the blood encounters at the level of the lungs, the blood shunts from the pulmonary artery to the aorta via the patent ductus arteriosus (PDA). Also, the increased pressure at the level of the RA favors the shunt from the RA to the left atrium (LA) via the patent foramen ovale (PFO) (see Fig. 11). Normally, high pulmonary vascular resistance together with low pressures at the level of the placenta are the factors that create higher rightsided pressure over systemic blood pressure in the fetus and therefore cause the shunt from right to left. Thus, the blood circulates from the pulmonary artery to the aorta via the PDA and from the RA to the left atrium (LA) via the foramen ovale.

The oxygenated blood goes from the LA to the LV to the aorta to oxygenate the heart, the brain, and the rest of the body tissues. Finally, the hypogastric arteries originate from the descending aorta. From there, the two umbilical arteries return nonoxygenated blood for exchange back to the placenta, exchanging CO_2 at the intervillous space for O_2. Then a new cycle of oxygenation will take place, and the umbilical vein will again carry oxygenated blood back to the fetus. This is the cycle of fetal circulation, and it shows the key role of the placenta in the process of fetal oxygenation.

In summary, shunting right to left is favored because of the increased pulmonary resistance and pressure over systemic pressure in fetal life. This is explained by the decreased resistance at the level of the placenta and the increased pulmonary vascular resistance. The best oxygenation is given to liver, heart, and brain.

At the time of birth, the expansion of the lungs decreases the pulmonary vascular resistance, and there is an increased blood flow to the lungs. Parallel to this, there is an increased pressure at the level of the umbilical vein because of the clamping of the umbilical cord. The improved blood flow at the level of the lungs will increase flow into the pulmonary vein, and the increased blood volume and pressure will reach the left atrium, closing the foramen ovale.

From the left atrium the blood flow goes to the left ventricle and then to the aorta. From the moment of birth, the systemic pressure will be higher than the pul-

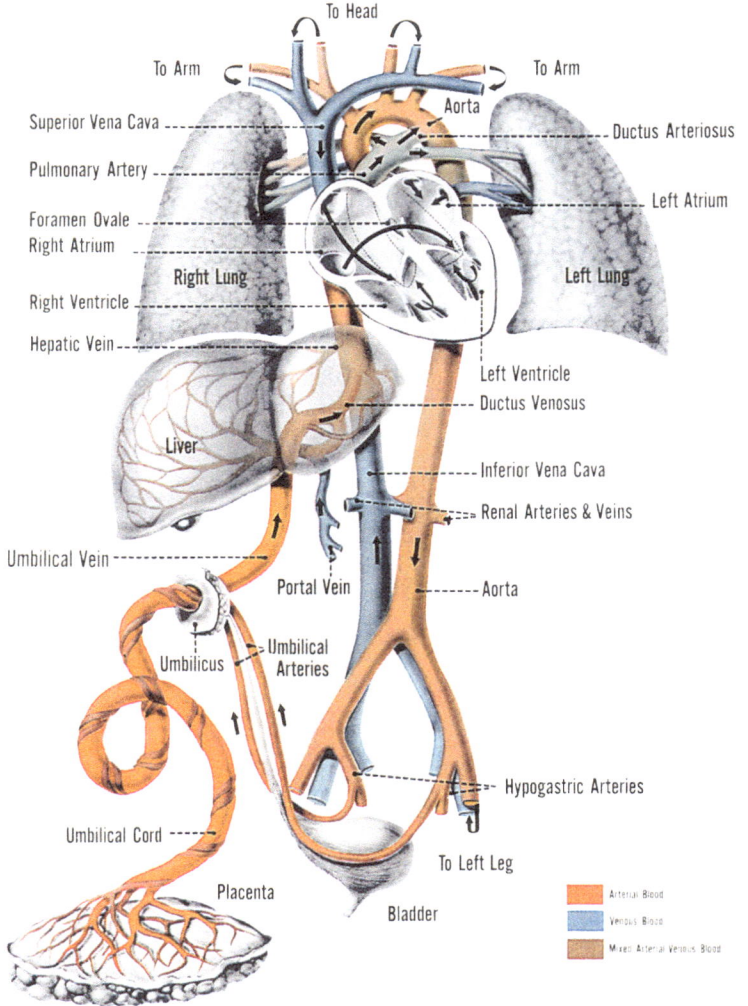

To Head

To Arm

To Arm

Aorta

Superior Vena Cava

Ductus Arteriosus

Pulmonary Artery

Left Atrium

Foramen Ovale
Right Atrium

Right Lung

Left Lung

Right Ventricle

Hepatic Vein

Left Ventricle

Ductus Venosus

Liver

Inferior Vena Cava

Renal Arteries & Veins

Umbilical Vein

Portal Vein

Aorta

Umbilicus

Umbilical
Arteries

Hypogastric Arteries

Umbilical Cord

To Left Leg

Placenta

Bladder

Arterial Blood

Venous Blood

Mixed Arterial Venous Blood

FIGURE 11. Fetal circulation. (Courtesy Ross Laboratories, © 1963.)

monary pressure if the adjustment in placenta and lung expansion takes place as expected. At birth the increased systemic pressure abolishes the right-to-left shunt through the PDA, and the ductus is obliterated. Thus, the normal pattern of oxygenation is established in the healthy newborn at the time of the first breath. At this moment, fetal circulation ends, and the pulmonary system of oxygenation takes over.

Knowing the stages of fetal oxygenation, the role of the placenta, and the details of the changeover to pulmonary oxygenation at birth is important in understanding the pathology of the mechanism of fetal oxygenation at birth should this transition not take place in the established order owing to maternal causes, placental dysfunction, or fetal causes, or a combination of them, causing fetal asphyxia.

12

Placental Insufficiency or Dysfunction

Placental insufficiency or dysfunction could be responsible for insufficient oxygenation during fetal life or at birth. Poor blood flow at the level of the placenta or poor perfusion may result in anoxia (lack of oxygenation) or ischemia (poor flow) or both, causing CO_2 retention and, if prolonged, metabolic acidosis.

At this stage of placental dysfunction at birth, prolonged hypoxia and ischemia can affect the baby. Under hypoxic stress, there is a redistribution of blood that will guarantee the best flow to the major organs—heart, brain, and adrenals—and diminished blood flow to limbs, gastrointestinal tract, and muscles.

The stress created by anoxia and ischemia eventually produces bradycardia and then circulatory collapse. Hypoxia at birth causes pulmonary vasoconstriction and increasing pulmonary vascular resistance, which explains asphyxia at birth.

Factors creating placental insufficiency at birth may include such systemic causes as hypertension, eclampsia, or convulsions in the mother, or uterine dystocias, insufficient uterine contractions with failure of labor to progress, placenta previa or abruptio placenta, cord around the neck, or prolapsed cord. These are frequent obstetric causes explaining fetal distress at birth because of hypoxia or ischemia and are reasons for perinatal asphyxia at this crucial stage of birth, causing brain asphyxia and circulatory failure.

Persistent Fetal Circulation

Placental dysfunction creates hypoxia, increases pulmonary vascular resistance, and can produce persistent fetal circulation (PFC), which is an expression of asphyxial stress at birth. PFC is characterized by asphyxia, which causes pulmonary vasoconstriction and pulmonary hypertension, leading to an overload of the right ventricle and heart failure.

In PFC there is a shunt from right to left because pulmonary pressures are higher than systemic pressures. Cyanosis is caused by a right-to-left shunt at the foramen ovale and ductal levels. There is respiratory distress and eventually heart failure and death unless the process can be reversed.

It therefore is important in a newborn with a history of fetal distress and who at birth presents with cyanosis, respiratory distress, and signs of congestive heart failure to consider PFC a likely diagnosis.

There are some characteristic features in the syn-

elevated PO_2 in blood obtained from the radial or temporal arteries in contrast with lower PO_2 in blood obtained from the abdominal aorta. This is because of reverse flow through the patent ductus into the descending aorta. Chest X ray shows increased bronchovascular markings as an expression of pulmonary congestion and increased pulmonary vascular resistance.

Right-to-left shunt is the dominant feature, explaining cyanosis, tachypnea, and congestive heart failure (CHF) with hepatomegaly as well as weak peripheral pulses. The ECG may show depression of the ST segments and low T waves compatible with myocardial ischemia. Echocardiography in PFC may reveal normal anatomic structures of the heart but right-to-left shunt through patent foramen ovale and/or ductus arteriosus. The right ventricle may contract poorly. The murmur is usually an expression of tricuspid insufficiency because of the enlarged size of the right ventricle. The right ventricle enlarges because of the increased pulmonary vascular resistance created by the nonexpanded lungs. This explains the increased venous pressure with right-to-left shunt and cyanosis. Progressive hypoxia and ischemia are the consequences. Poor flow to the left side of the heart favors ischemia of the main organs—heart and brain.

Summary of the Physiopathology of PFC

Hypoxia and ischemia may result from poor placental flow. This favors increased pulmonary vascular resistance, right-to-left shunting, cyanosis, and heart failure, as well as systemic hypoxia and ischemia because of poor flow and inadequate oxygenation in nonexpanded lungs

ETIOLOGY OF PERSISTENT FETAL CIRCULATION

Placental Dysfunction

Oxygen diminishes, which leads to retention of CO_2, H^+, and
acidosis

Hypoxic Ischemic Stress

There is redistribution of blood flow to the brain, heart, and
adrenals and a decrease in blood flow to lungs, limbs, and
gastrointestinal tract. Peripheral vasoconstriction leads to
bradycardia, hypertension, and cardiac failure or
circulatory collapse (shock)

PERSISTENT FETAL CIRCULATION IS A COMPLICATION OF:

Perinatal Asphyxia	Hypoxia
Leads to brain hypoxia and cardiac failure	Causes pulmonary vaso-constriction and pulmonary hypertension; this in-increases pulmonary vascular resistance

Persistent fetal circulation favors shunting right to left, causing
cyanosis and congestive heart failure.

FIGURE 12. Asphyxia creates placental deficiency during labor and
the prelabor period.

(Fig. 12). Arterial blood gases are better in the upper extremities than in the lower extremities, as are pulses.

This is a real contrast with the baby who up to birth
has normal placental function; well-oxygenated blood
from the uterine arterioles goes through the placental villi
to the umbilical vein, which carries fully oxygenated
blood to the fetus. This proper oxygenation will guarantee the transition of oxygenation from the placenta to the
automatically expanding lungs at birth. The cutting of
the umbilical cord and the expanding lungs favor good
flow to the lungs, so blood is then gradually oxygenated.
The good pulmonary flow provides adequate volume
and oxygenation to the pulmonary vein, filling the left
atrium, closing the foramen ovale, and filling the left
ventricle and aorta. From then on, systemic arterial pressures are higher than venous pressures, and the right-
to-left shunt is abolished through closure of the PDA and
foramen ovale.

Pink color of the newborn and good spontaneous
respirations are evidence that the transition of oxygenation from the placenta to the lungs took place in perfect harmony.

13

Fetal Breathing Movements

It has been documented both in animals and in humans that fetal breathing movements (FBM) exist *in utero* and that they may reflect the well-being or compromise of the fetus.

In animals the existence of FBM has been proved by measuring fetal intratracheal pressures. For this purpose a special catheter is used that is inserted into the trachea of fetal lambs. It records diaphragmatic movements by the use of an electromyogram as well as by registering fetal phrenic nerve activity.

In humans, for the last 10 years, studies have been done that documented the existence of FBM. With pressure-sensitive devices such as tocodynamometers and, lately, by ultrasonic A and B scans, it has been demonstrated that there are indeed FBM *in utero*.

These observations are well documented in term pregnancies (38–42 weeks of gestation) and are particularly useful during the last 2 weeks of gestation. It has also been proved that mutiparous mothers yield better recordings in this period of time.

FBM show a normal regular pattern when oxygen supply is adequate but may reflect hypoxia or asphyxia *in utero* when bradypnea, apnea, or a gasping pattern is documented. However, when 24-hr recordings are made, periods of pauses are seen to alternate with periods of normal breathing; these are also considered normal patterns and are called fetal sleeping periods.

When the fetus is under asphyxial stress, moderate or brief, the hypoxia produces bradypnea, documented by ultrasound, which may represent mild lack of oxygen (stage 1). If the lack of oxygen persists, then the FBM recording may show a progressive pattern of fetal distress; this will be reflected in bradypnea with periods of apnea (stage 2 or more severe degree of hypoxia). Finally, in the more severely compromised fetus with severe hypoxia or asphyxia, the fetal breathing will show a gasping pattern. This may represent a fetus under major asphyxial stress and therefore will reflect a life-threatening condition or risk of fetal death.

In summary, stage 1 is mild hypoxia causing bradypnea; stage 2 is prolonged or moderately severe hypoxia causing apnea; stage 3 is severe fetal asphyxia causing gasping.

It has been documented that changes in FBM can also be caused by nutritional, metabolic, or infectious disorders or multiple pregnancies. For example, studies done by Platt *et al.* in Los Angeles showed that AGA babies have a greater tendency to show a regular breathing pattern than SGA babies: fetal breathing movements were absent in 10 of 14 SGA babies (71%) but in only 10 of 122 AGA babies (7.9%) (Boddy and Dawes, 1976). Therefore, fetal nutrition or factors influencing fetal nutrition may play a significant role in fetal breathing.

We can conclude that AGA babies will have normal FBM patterns but that SGA, while *in utero*, may already show a compromised respiratory pattern (this was observed 2–4 weeks prior to delivery). Other factors such as intrauterine infections affecting the mother as well as the fetus may also cause changes in the FBM.

Metabolic causes such as diabetes in the mother may, because of hyperglycemia or fluctuations of blood sugar levels, cause changes in the FBM. Drugs, alcohol, and nicotine (in heavy-smoking mothers) may also produce changes, sometimes severe ones, in the FBM; this has been documented during the last period of pregnancy. Light anesthesia or sedation may cause depression in the FBM pattern.

It has also been demonstrated by Caldeyro-Barcia that fetal eupnea (normal FBM) can be related to normal fetal heart rate and that FBM showing different degrees of asphyxia, stage 2 (apnea) or stage 3 (gasping pattern), could correlate with more severe patterns of fetal deceleration.

The use of FBM to evaluate fetal well-being or fetal distress is a new tool for documenting babies at risk *in utero* even earlier than fetal deceleration, which, when present, is a sign of more progressive asphyxia and fetal compromise.

14

Adjustment in the Mechanism of Oxygenation at Birth

The newborn's condition at birth reflects how successful the changeover of the oxygenation process was. The first 5 min of life represent a crucial period of transition of oxygenation from the placenta to the infant's lungs. The child's future depends on successful adjustment in this crucial period.

Lack of oxygen during delivery will be reflected in the first 5 min of life in the appearance of the newborn and the manner of onset of his breathing.

The fetus enjoys a peaceful existence in the mother's uterus: the environment is hospitable, and he feels comfortable and warm, bathed by amniotic fluid; the placenta supplies nutrients from the mother and oxygen is provided by the umbilical vein of the cord.

From this very pleasant existence, the fetus is suddenly forced at 40 weeks or 9 months of gestation into a new environment. His chances for survival will no longer depend on the nutrition and oxygen supplied by the placenta but on the lungs' capacity to initiate breathing promptly, avoiding asphyxia. The crucial period during which the lungs must expand to guarantee oxygenation from the newborn's lungs is the first 5 min of life. Lack of oxygen before, during, or after delivery may result in asphyxia or death, or asphyxia of different degrees may lead to brain damage.

Apgar's excellent clinical summary lists the essential signs in the recognition of different degrees of oxygen deprivation (see Table 10). The Apgar score describes five elements in evaluation of a newborn at birth:

1. Color, from pink to blue (cyanosis).
2. Respirations, from spontaneous and regular to absent.
3. Cardiovascular, from good cardiac tones and frequency to slow heart rate (bradycardia).
4. Muscle tone, from active to limp.
5. Reaction to stimuli, from strong to nonreacting.

The Apgar score reflects the degree of oxygenation of the baby at birth.

Oxygen in good supply guarantees vitality and good performance in major systems, for example, lungs expanding well at birth, heart pumping well, and central nervous system active and commanding all basic neuromotor activities, which are reflected in the tone and spontaneous activity of the newborn. A well-oxygenated baby at birth reflects the changeover of oxygenation from the placenta to the lungs; thus, spontaneous breathing takes place promptly, assuring the continuation of life outside the uterus. The degrees of asphyxia from full oxygenation to oxygen compromise are represented in Table 11.

TABLE 10. Apgar Scores at Birth

	Healthy newborn		Sick newborn		Severely ill newborn	
Heart rate	>100	2	<100	1	50	1
Respiration	Strong Regular	2	Weak Irregular	1	Absent	0
Muscle tone	Active movement	2	Some flexion	1	Limp	0
Response to stimuli	Cry	2	Weak movements	1	None	0
Color	Pink	2	Pink body Blue extremities	1	Pale or blue	0
Apgar score		10		5		1

Group 1 represents the ideal newborn with a score of 10; a newborn with good vitality and oxygenation performs well:

1. Color is pink, score 2.
2. Respirations spontaneous and normal, score 2.
3. Cardiovascular: the heart beats with frequency of 120–160 beats/min, and the heart tones are of good quality, score 2.
4. Muscle tone active from birth and good spontaneous movements, score 2.
5. Reaction to stimuli: the newborn is alert and responds strongly to stimuli, score 2.

These five items score 2 each for a sum of 10, which represents top performance for a healthy newborn and a healthy start in life.

Group 2 represents the newborn who starts life with a moderate degree of asphyxia. This is reflected in changes in the following signs:

1. Color may show distal cyanosis but pink in the rest of the body, score 1.
2. Heart rate is normal, showing no compromise, score 2.
3. Respirations are spontaneous but not so regular, score 1.
4. Muscle tone may be normal or slightly diminished, score 1.
5. Reaction to stimuli is positive but not strong, score 1–2.

The total Apgar score of this baby will be 6–7, which reflects mild hypoxia.

If the asphyxia is more severe, then the Apgar score will be 5, showing a compromise in color with cyanosis more extensive, low tone, irregular slow breathing, slowing heart rate reflecting a more severe asphyxial stress, and poor reaction to stimuli. This newborn with an Apgar score of 5 reflects more severe asphyxial stress with central nervous system involvement.

Group 3 includes a newborn who is severely compromised. Asphyxia is severe and prolonged. Central nervous system involvement is reflected in this non-responsive newborn with flaccid tone, no respiratory effort, cyanotic color, and heart with severe bradycardia under 100 beats/min. The Apgar score is 1 or 2, reflecting some breathing effort and extreme bradycardia. This stage is incompatible with life: CNS damage is severe, as are the sequelae.

This stage represents severe asphyxia, metabolic acidosis, and brain impairment and is a very important cause of death in the perinatal period.

The Apgar score evaluates the newborn from the first to the fifth minute of life. If a depressed baby, when stimulated, responds by improved color, tone, and respiration in 5 min, the asphyxial stress is reversible, and improvement in the first to the fifth minute of life occurs. His prognosis may be good.

The unchanged low Apgar score represents a newborn with a progressive compromise in oxygenation and failure of adjustment as a result of the baby's make-up, maternal causes, obstetric complications, or a combination of these.

Asphyxia Type 3: Severe Asphyxia

This type of asphyxia produces a newborn who is severely compromised. Asphyxia is severe; there is no respiratory effort; the CNS is nonresponsive; the color is blue or cyanotic, indicating a lack of oxygen supply to all major systems. The heart rate is 50–100, and irregular heart beat is the last sign of life. Asphyxia type 3 is incompatible with life; if it is reversible, mortality and CNS damage are high. The leading cause of death in the perinatal period is asphyxia at birth.

The Transition from Intra- to Extrauterine Life in Normal Newborns

The Transition Period: Birth

At birth, the newborn moves from a warm liquid environment, the amniotic fluid, into the cold, dry delivery room. The umbilical vein ceases to be a source of placental oxygen, and the lungs, which had been nonfunctioning, now expand; the pulmonary circulation begins to function, and fetal circulation ceases. Removed from the soft, calm uterine environment, the newborn is now exposed to voices and instruments; from being untouched, he is suddenly handled, suctioned, and spanked, and his umbilical cord is clamped and cut. From darkness, he gets his first visual exposure to the world and his first look at his mother; this is the first "eye contact" period.

The Transition Continues: The First 24 Hours

The first period of extrauterine life, the first half hour, takes place in the delivery room. The newborn's color is pink, although there may be distal blue areas. The heart beats faster, 140–160 beats/min. Breathing is

TABLE 11. Degrees of Asphyxia at Birth

	Degree of asphyxia at birth		
System	Mild (type 1)[a]	Moderate (type 2)[b]	Severe (type 3)
Lungs	60–80 respirations per min	Irregular breathing Apnea	Apnea
Heart	Heart rate 120–160	Heart rate 100 or less	Heart rate irregular, < 100
CNS	Active movements	Flaccid	Nonresponsive Convulsions
Skin	Pink, distal cyanosis	Progressive cyanosis	Total cyanosis

[a]Newborn compensates for the asphyxia by breathing faster; heart is beating within normal frequency. Central nervous system is still active, as reflected in good muscle tone and spontaneous activity. Color shows mild cyanosis.
[b]Newborn is gradually compromised, or the asphyxia is more severe or prolonged. Heart rate is slowing; CNS is compromised, as shown in loss of muscle tone. Skin shows progressive cyanosis.

shallow, fast, and irregular, 40–50 breaths/min. Neurologically, the newborn is irritable and tremulous as a result of cold stress.

The second period, the next 2 hr, is spent in the
nursery. The newborn is completely pink. The heart has
slowed to 120 beats/min and is regular. Breathing, still
at 40–50 breaths/min, is regular. Neurologically, the baby
is more comfortable and shows normal movements with
no twitching.

The third period, hours 3 to 24 of life, are also spent
in the nursery. The vital signs are stable. The pulse is
120–160. Respiration is regular at 40–60/min. The color
is pink. Neurologically, there are normal movements and
no twitching or tremors, and the spontaneous sucking
reflex becomes apparent; the baby begins to suck.

Adjustment of the Different Systems at Birth

The respiratory system changes from placental to
pulmonary oxygen. This adjustment is easier in babies
who are head presentations, a position which favors the
expulsion of fluids from the lungs and thus aids lung expansion, than in breech presentations or cesarean sec-
tions performed because of breech presentations.

As the lungs expand at birth, circulation in the lungs
improves, as does oxygen flow, and the diminished lung
resistance favors blood flow. This increases pressure in
the left side of the heart and favors the closing of the patent ductus arteriosus and the foramen ovale.

As oxygenation by the lungs is established, oxygenation of the major organs improves. The increased oxygen supply stimulates brain performance, and improved

supplies of calcium, sugar, and electrolytes provide metabolic balance and make the adjustment period easier.

Renal flow improves parallel to the improvement of heart and lung circulation, and renal vascular resistance diminishes to normal. Blood pressure is stable, and kidney function is gradually established to maintain homeostasis (equilibrium between electrolytes and proteins).

The liver is the great center of blood formation in uterine life from 2 to 6 months of gestation; bilirubin exchange during intrauterine life is performed by the placenta. After birth, the liver enzyme glucuronyl transferase is responsible for the conversion of bilirubin from indirect to direct, and direct bilirubin is then excreted by the kidneys. Transient insufficiency of this enzyme, together with renal factors such as immature function, explains the possibility of so-called physiological jaundice.

Cold stress at birth can be very damaging for the newborn. Cold stress increases oxygen consumption and oxygen requirements and increases energy production and heat loss. The baby adjusts by increasing metabolic lactose production, and metabolic acidosis is the end result of this stress.

Cold stress produces vasoconstriction to avoid heat loss and creates diminishing blood flow to peripheral areas which leads to tissue hypoxia (or lack of oxygen), resulting in pallor followed by cyanosis (blue color of the extremities). This situation is more dangerous in the small newborn, SGA, or premature, where the termoregulation mechanism is not mature; therefore, cold stress is more difficult to adjust to and control in the small infant at birth.

Care Given to the Baby in the Delivery Room

The most important crucial steps in taking care of a newborn are the following:

1. To stimulate breathing.
2. To receive the baby in a warm environment and avoid cold exposure.
3. To welcome the newborn in an environment free from infection. Ensuring adequate breathing and warming and a sterile environment are the essential elements in caring for a newborn baby in the delivery room. Thus, immediately after the delivery of the head, the baby is suctioned to clear the nose and mouth of secretions and enable immediate breathing.
4. The umbilical cord is clamped, usually in about 2 min. The baby is put in a position lower than the mother's body to allow a flow of blood from the umbilical cord and the placenta. In these 2 min a blood volume of about 100 ml enters the newborn, representing an extra amount of blood and furnishing an extra amount of oxygen until the lungs fully expand to assure the baby's breathing. After the cord is clamped, the baby is wrapped and kept warm and comfortable.
5. The Apgar scores in the first minute and at 3 and 5 min are determined to evaluate the degree of oxygenation as well as the baby's vitality. At this time if the Apgar score is 9 to 10, this healthy newborn is wrapped and given to the mother. This immediate exposure is psychologically very important to the mother. After the baby is actually held by the mother, he is given to the nurse for further care.

6. The eyes are cleared by eye drops, either antibiotics or silver nitrate, a classical antiseptic, to avoid infection of the eyes or ophthalmia neonatorum.
7. Vitamin K (1 mg) is given i.m. to prevent hemorrhagic disease of the newborn.
8. A rapid evaluation in the delivery room includes, in addition to the Apgar scores at 1, 3, and 5 min, the general vitality of the newborn and examination for any anomalies of head, neck, chest, or hip, or any other orthopedic anomalies.

Thus concludes the first stage in the life of the newborn baby.

15

Birth Asphyxia in the Full-Term Infant

Some of the factors causing asphyxia at birth are described in detail in Chapter 17 on high-risk infants (HRI), but it is important to be aware of the causes that may compromise oxygenation in full-term babies:

1. Prolonged labor.
2. Cephalopelvic disproportion.
3. Mother's exhaustion during labor.
4. Cord around the neck, a frequent cause of asphyxia during delivery.
5. Difficulties in delivery such as breech presentations.
6. Trauma of birth in large babies.
7. Eclampsia.
8. Placenta previa.
9. Abruptio placenta.
10. Syndrome of meconium aspiration.

Meconium aspiration is one of the most traumatic complications causing severe asphyxia in full-term babies. Full details of this syndrome are described in Chapter 17.

Mechanisms of Lung Expansion at Birth in Full-Term Babies and a Normal Newborn

The mechanisms of lung expansion at birth are the following:

1. Chest compression of the newborn at labor and delivery. Sometimes these compressions are equivalent to 20 to 30 or occasionally 60 cm H_2O.
2. The clamping of the umbilical cord.
3. A transient cold stress (changing temperatures from the uterus to the temperature of the delivery room).
4. The accumulation of CO_2, which stimulates receptors (neck receptors) of the newborn that may affect the respiratory centers of the brain responsible for initiating respirations.

In a normal full-term pregnancy and a normal spontaneous delivery, the stages of delivery cause no stress on the newborn baby, since he is anatomically and functionally prepared. The mature newborn has a consistent chest, good muscle tone development, and mature lungs able to expand well with enough surfactant to help the bronchial alveolar space resist collapse, and an active and intact central nervous system to initiate breathing. In addition, this newborn has a good heart that maintains circulation. All these factors reflect the fact that this baby is the offspring of a normal pregnancy and delivery and

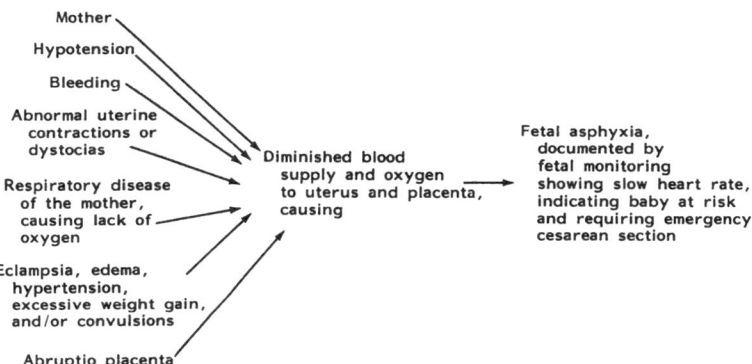

FIGURE 13. Factors affecting pregnancy at delivery that cause fetal asphyxia.

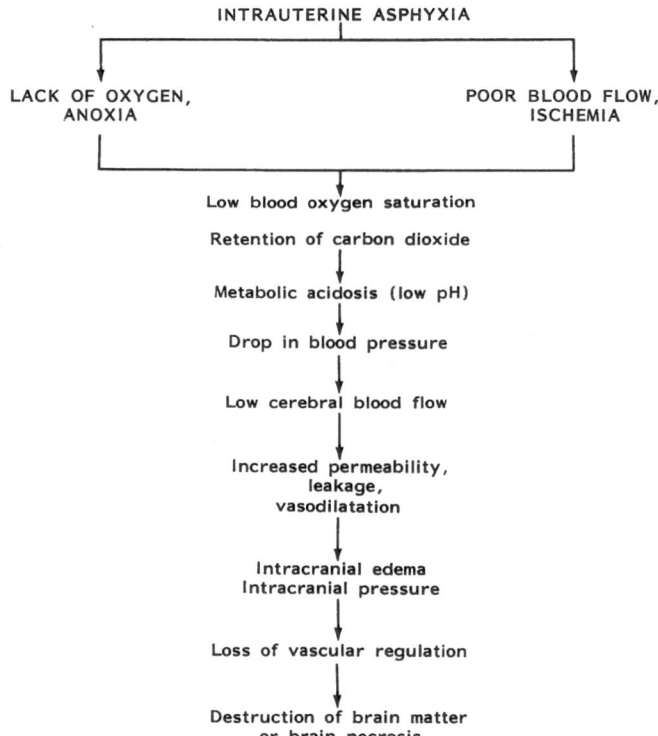

FIGURE 14. Causes of fetal brain damage.

has adjusted well to extrauterine life in the crucial first 5 min of life.

On the other hand, the baby with a low Apgar score of 5 or less at birth, with poor color, slow heartbeat, poor to limp muscle tone, and failure to react to stimuli, represents a newborn with severe asphyxial compromise. This baby's life prognosis is guarded (see Figs. 13 and 14).

16

Detecting Fetal Distress

Fetal distress represents fetal asphyxia or lack of oxygen. Fetal distress during labor can be detected by fetal monitoring. Electrodes are applied on the mother's abdomen and will detect fetal distress as slowing of the fetal heart rate.

A fetal heart rate of under 100, if maintained for more than 3 to 5 min independent of uterine contractions (variable decelerations, Dips III according to Caldeyro-Barcia), means that the baby is poorly oxygenated and under a severe asphyxial stress. This baby should be immediately delivered by cesarean section to avoid the progressive damage of asphyxia.

This baby when delivered will have an Apgar score of 5, namely, 1 for color, 1 for slow heartbeat, 1 for irregular breathing, 1 for low to limp muscle tone, and 1 for poor reaction to stimuli. This baby is a compromised baby reflecting at birth the stress of asphyxia.

In the depressed baby, oxygen and intravenous fluid therapy to correct metabolic acidosis and other metabolic changes are essential to restore a normal pattern of life. The survival of this compromised baby will depend on the speed of care, the quality of the equipment, as well as the skills of the professional who is providing acute care in the neonatal ICU to this newborn.

From the descriptions in this and the preceding chapter, it is obvious that the vitality shown in these two groups of babies in the first 5 min of life is quite different. Also different are the prognosis and the future of these two lives.

Thus, the first 5 min of life in a newborn may reflect a healthy start or a compromised one. The baby with an Apgar score of 10 may have a normal life, normal development, and normal milestones. The baby with significant asphyxial distress at birth and an Apgar score of 5 or less will be affected by central nervous system compromise resulting in degrees of neuromotor or psychoneuromotor impairment from cerebral palsy to different degrees of developmental delay in motor, intellectual, or lingual compromise reflecting different degrees of minimal brain dysfunction.

17

Asphyxia in the High-Risk Infant

It has been documented that 10% of total births suffer from some degree of asphyxia. It has also been shown by recording fetal breathing movements that small-for-gestational-age (SGA) infants and very-low-birth-weight (VLBW) infants suffer different degrees of asphyxia *in utero* even 2 to 4 weeks prior to delivery, showing bradypnea, apnea, and a gasping pattern that reflect, respectively, mild to severe asphyxia. This chapter discusses the many factors that affect the mechanism of asphyxial stress in the group of high-risk babies.

Evaluation of the High-Risk Infant in the Perinatal Period

The perinatal period represents the first 7 days of life. The clinical appearance of the high-risk infant is reflected in the following clinical indices:

1. Color from pale to cyanotic (blue color).
2. Respirations irregular, rapid, with progressive respiratory distress, grunting, flaring, and intercostal and subcostal retractions.
3. Central nervous system symptoms: depression, muscle tone flaccid or diminished, progressive irritability, tremors, and convulsions.
4. Head appearance: the size of the head, the tension of the anterior fontanelle, signs of trauma, bruises, and hematomas are all important observations.

These four indices precede the next stage, which includes asphyxia or inadequate brain oxygenation, thus explaining irritability followed by depression and finally convulsions and coma.

The causes of the serious condition of this newborn are trauma, infection, hemorrhage, metabolic problems, and asphyxia. All are common stress factors in the adaptation to extrauterine life. However the form of the reaction will depend greatly on the make-up of the baby. Therefore, this chapter considers the high-risk baby in five groups.

Group 1: Adequate for Gestational Age

This newborn infant is the product of a normal pregnancy. The height and weight at birth correspond to those found at term pregnancy (38 to 42 weeks). The birth weight of the AGA baby at term will range between 2800 and 3800 g (7 to 8.3 lb); the height will be from 46 to 51 cm (18 to 20.5 inches); the head circumference will be 32 to 35 cm (12.8 to 14 inches). These values represent the range from 10% to 90%. The term newborn whose height, weight, and head circumference values are within these ranges is AGA for a 38- to 42-week baby.

If an AGA baby presents at birth with an abnormality of color, respiration, or central nervous system, the cause is related to the period of birth immediately before or immediately after labor. The most frequent causes are asphyxia at birth, trauma or aspiration of amniotic fluid post- or intrapartum, or sometimes, in depressed babies, sedation analgesia or anesthesia given to the mother.

The pathology associated with the above symptoms in an AGA baby is related to the birth period (see Tables 12 and 13).

Group 2: Small for Gestational Age

The baby's height, weight, and head circumference are below the tenth percentile at birth, e.g., 2500 g, 45 cm, and 31 cm, respectively. Clinically, the baby shows pallor, irregular breathing with signs of respiratory distress, flaccidity, tremors or convulsions, and a small head. These symptoms in the SGA newborn result from factors such as the following:

1. Inadequate nutrition in the mother during pregnancy.
2. Intrauterine infection before (not during) labor, which may interfere with intrauterine growth: toxoplasmosis, rubella, cytomegalovirus, and herpes (TORCH) as documented by antibody titers.
3. Drugs used by the mother.

In this SGA newborn, the serious condition at birth results from a combination of intrauterine problems and risks at birth.

Group 3: Large for Gestational Age

This is the baby who, at birth, has values of weight, height, and head circumference above the 90th percentile, e.g., 4000 g, 53 cm, and 36 cm, respectively. This type of newborn (LGA) will also reflect distress in color (pale to blue), respiratory distress, and twitching or convulsions. The baby's symptoms represent a double pathology: metabolic stress during pregnancy and stress of labor and delivery.

A typical example of the LGA baby is the offspring of a diabetic mother. These babies are always LGA, always hypoglycemic, and susceptible to weight loss. They develop twitching or convulsions because of low blood sugar. Because of their large size at birth, they are at risk for trauma, asphyxia, and metabolic problems.

The pathology of the LGA baby is a combination of prenatal factors (metabolic, diabetes of the mother) and genetic and birth trauma.

Group 4: Intrauterine Growth Retardation

This is an example of a baby not only SGA but also showing remarkable developmental delays in weight and height values and a very small head circumference (see Table 14). His risks at birth are reflected in his color (pale to blue), varying degrees of respiratory distress, and CNS signs (flaccidity, depression, tremors, or convulsions). These are all signs of a newborn showing severe compromise in intrauterine growth and aggravated by the stress of birth, for which he has poor tolerance.

Causes in this group include intrauterine virus infections, nutritional factors, drugs, and nicotine (smoking mother). These babies may present with congenital anomalies.

Group 5: Very Low Birth Weight

This group of babies was considered nonviable a decade ago. Its survival represents a triumph of perinatology since 1975. Included in this group is the premature, immature infant whose gestational age ranges from 28 to 32 weeks and whose birth weight is under 1200 g. This is a high-risk baby because of the total immaturity of all of his systems, in particular the respiratory and central nervous systems. The lungs are immature and unable to breathe. The CNS is also immature in regulating breathing and is susceptible to bleeding (brain hemorrhage). The kidneys are immature and subject to infections.

These babies require assisted ventilation in order to breathe, which increases the risk of brain hemorrhage and respiratory arrest from the increased pressure. Irregular heartbeats, episodes of flaccidity, pallor or cyanosis, and convulsions are constant risks.

Causes in this group include immature systems, congenital anomalies, and the risk of brain hemorrhage complicated by the trauma of birth and asphyxia (see Table 15, Figs. 15–17).

TABLE 12. High-Risk Infants: Causes and Clinical Appearance

	AGA	SGA	LGA	IUGR	VLBW
Clinical	Height, weight, and head circumference between 10 and 90%	Height, weight, and HC under 10%	Height, weight, and HC above 90%	Mature but very SGA	Gestation 28-32 weeks
	Term newborn Wt: 2800–3800 g Ht: 46–51 cm HC: 32–35 cm	Term newborn Wt: <2500 g Ht: 45 cm HC: 31 cm	Term newborn Wt: >4 kg Ht: >53 cm HC: >36 cm	Extreme SGA	Weight <1200 g
Color	Pale Blue (cyanosis) Meconium stained	Pale to blue	Pale to blue	Pale to blue Jaundice	Pale to blue Bruises
Respirations	Irregular, fast Respiratory distress	Irregular, fast Respiratory distress	Irregular, fast Respiratory distress	Irregular, fast Respiratory distress	Irregular, fast Hyaline membrane disease

Cry	Weak	Weak	Weak	Weak	Weak
Tone	Low to limp	Low to limp	Low to twitch Convulsions	Low to twitching	Low Twitching Convulsions
Head	Molding Hematomas Anterior fontanelle full	Small	Large Anterior fontanelle full	Small	Small hematomas
Causes	Asphyxia Trauma Aspiration Infection Oversedation of mother	Nutrition Intrauterine infections Drugs	Metabolic Diabetic mother Trauma Asphyxia	Intrauterine infections Nutrition Alcohol Drugs Nicotine	Immature systems Brain bleeding Congenital anomalies
Pathology	Birth period	Pregnancy to labor	Pregnancy and labor	Pregnancy and labor Congenital anomalies	Pregnancy Birth trauma Asphyxia Hemorrhage

TABLE 13. Effects of Postmaturity and Dysmaturity on Infants at Risk

	Postmature	Dysmature
Cause	Postterm pregnancy	Placenta dysfunction
Gestational age	More than 42 weeks of gestation	Less than 40 weeks of gestation (SGA)
Skin	Dry, peeling, stained Long nails	Peeling, looks immature
Looks	Alert, open eyes	Immature
Weight	More than 3 kg Weight loss	Less than 2500 g
Height	More than 20 inches (50 cm), taller than average full-term newborn	Less than 20 inches
Pathology	Postdue Aging placenta	Diseased placenta or general disease Placenta dysfunction or insufficiency: small, fibrotic Systemic causes: Infections Nutrition Alcohol Cigarettes

Grade, clinical appearance	Stage I: looks healthy, open eyes, mature, nutrition wasted, signs of weight loss Stage II: asphyxia, risk of respiratory distress (if not delivered) Stage III: meconium aspiration (if not delivered)	High-risk baby Respiratory problems Metabolic: low on Ca and sugar Infections
Complications	If more than 42 weeks, wasting, nutrition impaired Weight loss Asphyxia Aspiration pneumonia	Respiratory infections Asphyxia Metabolic problems: acidosis, low sugar (hypoglycemia), low calcium (hypocalcemia)

TABLE 14. Intrauterine Infections Causing IUGR:
Symptoms, Outcome, and Treatment

Disease	Cause	Transmission	Clinical appearance	Type of baby	Outcome	Comments	Treatment and diagnosis
Rubella	Virus	Transplacental	Microcephaly Cataracts Heart disease Deafness Gregg syndrome	IUGR SGA	Serious under 8 weeks of gestation	Baby may shed virus for 1 year; nursing personnel should have rubella titers	Treatment of sequelae in the baby; rubella vaccine prior to pregnancy; TORCH titers
Herpes	Virus	Transplacental Congenital Type I: oral and skin lesion Type II: neonatal herpes genitalis	Microcephaly Brain calcification Skin lesions Type II: fulminant infection	IUGR SGA AGA	CNS damage High mortality	Cesarean section for herpes II	Arabinoside in baby i.v. TORCH titers + for herpes

Cytomegalovirus	Virus	Transplacental, respiratory route, or venereal	Microcephaly Small eyes Hepatitis Enlarged liver and spleen	IUGR SGA	CNS and vision damage	Severe in gestation less than 8 weeks	TORCH + Infant is infective via saliva and urine No specific therapy
Toxoplasmosis	*Toxoplasma gondi*	Eating undercooked pork Transplacental	Microcephaly Chorioretinitis Hepatitis Enlarged liver and spleen Jaundice	IUGR SGA	CNS and vision damage	Avoid eating raw pork	Daraprin in adults TORCH + for *Toxoplasma* titers
Syphilis	*Treponema pallidum*	Sexual transmission Transplacental	Sanguinolent rhinitis Skin lesions: mouth, anus CNS lesions Osteochondritis	AGA SGA	CNS damage Bone lesions	Serology in all prospective mothers	Penicillin to mother and baby

[a]Gregg syndrome leads to microcephaly, cataracts, heart disease, and deafness. It is caused by rubella virus in the first 3 months of pregnancy.

TABLE 15. Conditions Associated with IUGR, VLBW, and SGA:
Prognosis and Treatment

Condition	Diagnosis	Treatment	Prognosis
HMD	Chest X ray	Oxygen Assisted respiration IPPV	Improved
IVH, severe asphyxia	32 weeks Less than 1200 g Sonogram, CAT scan Hydrocephalus	VPS (ventricular peritoneal shunt) for hydrocephalus	Improved
Hypoxia	Low Apgar Twitching A&B	Physical therapy Oxygen IPPB	Paresis Diplegia Partial recovery
IUGR	Sonogram, TORCH titers during pregnancy	Physical therapy Supportive Oxygen	Improved
SGA	High-risk pregnancy	Treat high-risk pregnancy for prophylaxis of SGA	MBD Seizures
Congenital anomalies, chromosomal	Amniocentesis α-Fetoproteins	End pregnancy	Severe sequelae

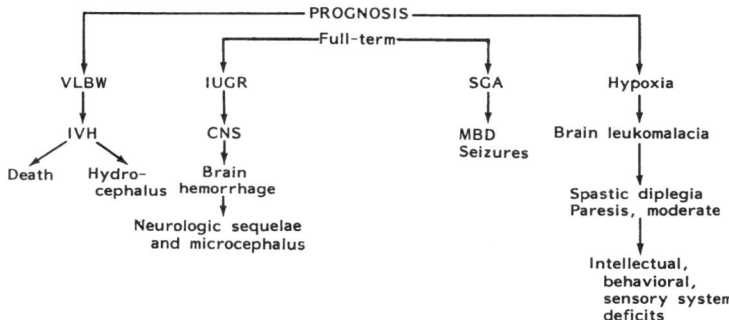

FIGURE 15. Immediate and late complications of hypoxia and anoxia in the newborn.

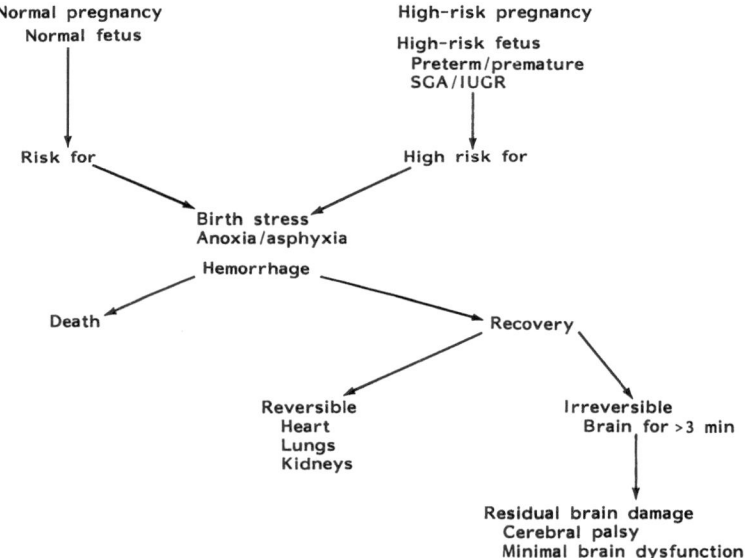

FIGURE 16. Immediate and late outcomes for the high-risk infant.

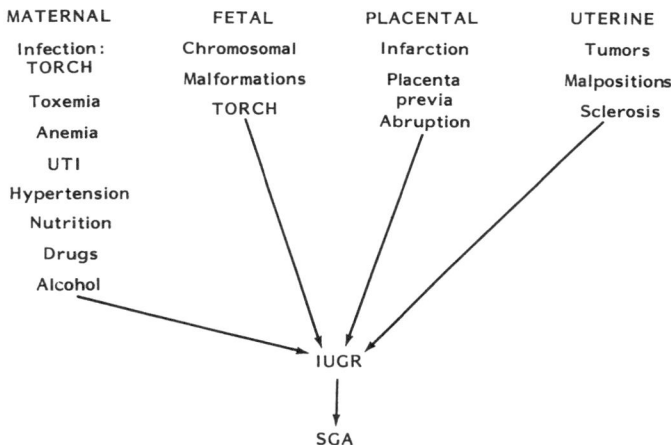

FIGURE 17. Causes of intrauterine growth retardation. A useful method used today is sonography, which can detect IUGR. Delivery of the baby will be justified after 37 weeks if IUGR is documented. The sonographic measurements used are head circumference, abdomen circumference, and length of femur in relation to the gestational age.

18

Monitoring High-Risk Infants

In the last decade great advances were made in perinatology, which evaluates fetal growth from 26 weeks of gestation to the end of the neonatal period or the fourth week after birth. The new techniques used in perinatology in recent years include amniocentesis. Evaluation of the amniotic fluid by this technique makes it possible to detect changes and to diagnose chromosomal abnormalities including different types of trisomies. This technique may also reveal the presence of abnormal substances such as α-fetoprotein, which often predicts the risk of malformations such as spina bifida and meningoceles. Also, the evaluation of fetomaternal hormones such as estriol in blood or urine may confirm fetal well-being or detect fetal risk. For example, urine estriol levels of 12 mg collected in 24 hr reveal fetal well-being, whereas levels of 4 mg may detect a fetus at risk (Fig. 18; Table 16).

Fetal monitoring, an electronic technique, may detect a fetus at risk by recording fetal heart rate. Fetal deceleration representing stress and asphyxia is documented by fetal monitoring.

Sonography to determine gestational age		Amniocentesis to determine lung maturity		Estriol levels to determine fetal well-being	
BPD 8.8	BPD 9.5	L/S 1.49	L/S 2	4 mg	12 mg
Risk	No risk	Risk	No risk	Risk	No risk

Fetal monitoring: Depressions

Early	Late	Variable
FHR < 100 at beginning of contraction	FHR < 100 at end of contraction	Deceleration at any time
Risk	Major risk	More risk
	Poor prognosis	

FIGURE 18. Procedures used to document high-risk babies and their prognosis. BPD, biparietal diameter; L/S, lecithin-sphingomyelin ratio; FHR, fetal heart rate; UC, uterine contraction.

TABLE 16. Fetal Heart Rate Changes
as Indications of Fetal Distress

Fetal acceleration (to heart rate >160)
  Maternal emotional stress, anxiety
  Hypotension
  Fever
  Infection
  Hyperthyroidism
  Early stage of fetal asphyxia
Fetal deceleration, early (to heart rate <120 during uterine contractions)
  Anesthesia: spinal or caudal
  Mechanical compression of umbilical cord
    [change position of mother to left lateral][a]
  Oxytocin therapy causing uterine contractions
    [discontinue i.v. oxytocin]
  Cord around neck of fetus
    [maneuver to release cord]
  Prolapsed cord as presenting part at delivery
    [maneuver to reposition cord; otherwise cesarean]
  Maternal hypotension
    [increase i.v. infusion and elevate legs]
  Prognosis is good if cause is treated and asphyxia is reversible
Fetal deceleration, late or prolonged (represents severe asphyxia)
  Maternal hypertension
  Preeclampsia
  Diabetes
  Intrauterine infections causing IUGR
  Maternal age (old primigravida)
  Prognosis is reserved for the fetus because prolonged decelerations rep-
    resent prolonged fetal asphyxia; a heart rate <70 for >30 sec is a
    severe deceleration

---

[a]Treatments of the indicated causes are indicated in brackets.

Sonography permits the diagnosis of fetal growth and the degree of fetal maturity and can document abnormalities of fetal size, head, or skeleton.

All these techniques together, when indicated, can provide information about babies who are potentially at risk. Measurement of the bitemporoparietal diameter of the fetus by the use of sonography is a valuable technique in the assessment of fetal age and fetal growth. For example, a bitemporoparietal diameter of 8.8 cm in a fetus indicates that the fetus is at 35 weeks of gestation, whereas a diameter of 9.5 cm will indicate that the fetus is at term or 38 to 42 weeks.

By evaluating amniotic fluid obtained by amniocentesis, it is possible to determine the presence of two phopholipids, lecithin and sphingomyelin (L,S). When the L/S ratio exceeds 2, the lungs of the fetus are mature enough to permit breathing. However, if the L/S ratio is less than 2, this newborn baby risks the development of hyaline membrane disease (HMD) because his lungs are immature.

Simultaneous recordings are made of the fetal heart rate (FHR) and uterine contractions, and variations from certain standards may reflect fetal risk or fetal asphyxia. For example, a fetal heart rate of more than 160 for more than 10 min is fetal distress; maternal causes may be fever, anxiety, infection, or hyperthyroidism. A fetal heart rate of 100 or less following uterine contractions or independent of them represents late or variable deceleration, Dips II or III, and this is equivalent to moderate to severe fetal asphyxia.

Early deceleration is the slowing of the fetal heart rate at the beginning of the uterine contraction. The cause of this slowing of the fetal heart rate is compression of the fetal head resulting from uterine contractions. Seldom does the FHR go under 100.

Late deceleration is the slowing of the fetal heart rate at the peak of the uterine contraction and even extending to after the contraction is over.

Variable deceleration can be defined as a type of deceleration that may be observed at any time during labor, not necessarily related to uterine contractions, lasting seconds or minutes.

Caldeyro-Barcia recommends that even early decelerations require a thorough follow-up of these babies after delivery to determine psychoneuromotor potential and limitations because of the risk of asphyxia at birth (reflected by fetal deceleration) and its implications for the neuromotor development of this type of infant.

In summary, early decelerations (Dips I) are caused by head compression, late decelerations (Dips II) are caused by placental dysfunction, and variable decelerations (Dips III) are caused by prolonged cord compression with resultant asphyxia and metabolic acidosis.

19

Obstetric and Medical Intervention

Obstetric Interference

Much of the material discussed in this chapter is based on the pioneering work of Caldeyro-Barcia (1975), who originated much of today's technology for fetal monitoring. Caldeyro-Barcia stresses three possible sources of intrapartum risk to the newborn (Table 17):

1. The risk of early rupture of membranes (ROM).
2. Inadequate use of oxytocin to stimulate uterine contraction.
3. The position of the mother during labor.

He further emphasizes the importance of obstetric intervention during labor. Early rupture of membranes causes an increase in pressure over the fetal head as well as compression of the umbilical cord, which can lead to asphyxia and brain hemorrhage.

TABLE 17. Obstetric Interference with
Amniotic Membranes during Delivery

Rupture of membranes	Spontaneous rupture (SRM)	Rupture at 4 cm of dilatation (ERM)
Pressure of the uterine contractions over skull	Symmetrical	Asymmetric
Malalignment frontoparietal–occipital	No	Yes
Fetal deceleration	No	Yes
Uterine contractions causing compression over head and umbilical cord	Symmetrical	Asymmetric
EEG of the fetus during delivery and at birth	Normal	Epileptic changes
Skull X ray	Normal to 34% malalignment	Abnormal; 50% malalignment
Rupture of the tentorium	No	Yes
Brain hemorrhage	No	Yes
Perinatal deaths caused by brain hemorrhage (first week of life)	0%	30%
Caput succedaneum (the accumulation of interstitial fluid under the scalp)	5%	15%
Subdural hemorrhage	No	Yes
Duration of labor from 4 to 10 cm dilatation	180 min	126 min
Neurological examination	Normal	Abnormal (because of brain trauma)
EEG changes	Normal, no changes	Abnormal EEG from 1 to 100 days after birth

Maintenance of intact amniotic membranes until the end of labor is important to protect the fetal head from compression by uterine contractions and to prevent misalignment of the skull bones, which can tear the meningeal plexus and lead to hemorrhagic complications.

The first stage of labor lasts 11–15 hr, and cervical dilatation reaches 3–4 cm. Caldeyro-Barcia studied two groups of newborns: in one group, there was early rupture of the membranes (ERM); in the other, there was spontaneous rupture of the membranes (SRM) at the end of the first stage of labor. The total time for delivery was 126 min in the ERM group versus 180 min in the SRM group, a difference of over 50 min. The two groups also differed with respect to incidence of skull deformities, fetal decelerations, brain trauma, asphyxiation, and hemorrhage. Incidence of caput succedaneum was 15% among ERM and 5% among SRM babies. Further, in ERM, the heart rate dropped from 150 to 110 at the time of the membrane rupture. Recordings of EEGs at the time of birth were normal in the SRM group but showed epileptiform characteristics in the ERM group. Similarly, results of neurological examinations at birth were normal among SRM babies and abnormal among ERM babies. On the basis of these findings, Caldeyro-Barcia considers it unjustified to attempt to hasten delivery of SRM babies, which would expose them to risks of head trauma, asphyxia, and hemorrhage.

Finally, Caldeyro-Barcia's studies have shown that the supine position should be avoided by the mother at the time of delivery because this position causes compression of the descending aorta and inferior vena cava and can produce fetal asphyxia. Caldeyro-Barcia found that the fetal pulse slows while the mother rests on her back and immediately accelerates when she assumes a prone position or rests on her left side. Further, Caldeyro-Barcia recommends walking during the period of cervical dilatation.

Medical Intervention and Interference

Over the last 15 years, new techniques have been developed to evaluate high-risk pregnancies and to induce labor and delivery. This section discusses pharmacological agents and tests, the evaluation of high-risk pregnancies, and fetal risk.

The Use of Oxytocin

Oxytocin is a hormone secreted by the posterior pituitary gland that stimulates labor. It increases uterine contractility. When synthetic oxytocin is infused intravenously, uterine contractions start, and their strength depends on the quantity of oxytocin given. Caldeyro-Barcia states that only 2% of labors require oxytocin but that it has been used in more than 40% of deliveries. Its effectiveness in stimulating uterine contraction is about 85%, but there are risks because excessive contractions may cause pressure on the fetal head or compression of the cord, leading to asphyxia.

Rupture of Membranes

Rupture of membranes in the first stage of labor (3- to 4-cm dilatation) to speed labor may cause risks and expose the fetus to serious hazards. Normally, when the amniotic sac is intact until the end of labor, the pressures of each uterine contraction pass wavelike over the fetus. When the amniotic sac is ruptured, amniotic fluid no longer protects the fetal head, and strong contractions may have a traumatic effect. Increased uterine contractions may cause rupture of the uterus or early separation of the placenta (abruptio placenta), creating the risk of bleeding and severe distress for both mother and fetus.

Therefore, early rupture of the membranes is only justified as an emergency procedure and should not be used simply to speed delivery.

Oxytocin Challenge Test

The oxytocin challenge test (OCT) has been used in conjunction with electronic fetal monitoring (EFM) to detect pregnancies at risk from 32 to 44 weeks of gestation. The test consists of infusing intravenous oxytocin and recording the fetal heart rate by EFM. A decrease in the fetal heart rate to 100 or less without recovery to a normal 120–140 between contractions indicates fetal distress.

Electronic Fetal Monitoring

Electronic fetal monitoring was developed by Caldeyro-Barcia and has been widely used to detect high-risk babies.

In external EFM, electrodes are applied to the mother's abdomen, and the fetal heart rate is recorded to detect fetal distress. External EFM can be carried out in conjunction with monitoring of the intensity of uterine contractions so that these can be correlated with changes in the fetal heart rate. In addition, ultrasound has been used to detect fetal activity while the other measurements are being made.

Internal EFM is used only in high-risk pregnancies. In internal EFM, one electrode is applied to the mother's abdomen, and a second electrode is applied directly to the scalp of the fetus after rupture of membranes and dilatation to 3–4 cm. Because of the risks associated with rupture of the membranes and application of an electrode to the fetal scalp *in utero,* internal EFM is justified only in high-risk pregnancies.

20

Follow-up of the Asphyxiated Infant

The follow-up of the asphyxiated baby presents a medical challenge regarding the potential for and limitations of future handicaps. Asphyxia if prolonged represents a multiple risk in which trauma, metabolic disorders, and infection are factors added to the initial asphyxial–ischemic damage. Asphyxia also adds extra risks such as bleeding to the immature brain of the VLBW or SGA infant who, because of intrauterine factors (nutrition, drugs, or intrauterine infections), is more susceptible to the asphyxial stress of birth.

In addition, the LGA baby, in addition to the metabolic problem of being the offspring of a diabetic mother, is subject to the traumatic and asphyxial stress of delivery of a large infant.

This chapter discusses the baby's follow-up, his potentials and limitations, as well as the tests used to determine his degree of development.

After Discharge

In the premature newborn infant of less than 1500 g (3.1 lb), follow-up is required to observe, diagnose, and treat any type of psychoneuromotor deficits as he grows older.

The causes that may lead to compromise of the central nervous system as he grows older are usually related to immaturity of the brain and risks at birth or shortly after. These include:

1. Asphyxia.
2. Brain hemorrhage.
3. Infection.
4. Metabolic problems.
5. Jaundice.
6. Trauma.

Major risks are observed in the group weighing less than 1200 g (2.6 lb) with low Apgar scores at birth (5 or under) at 1 and 5 min of life. These babies have a high risk of brain hemorrhage aggravated by hyaline membrane disease, and lung immaturity requiring assisted or controlled ventilation by the use of mechanical ventilators.

After the vital risk is over and central nervous system functions are stable and respiratory, infection, and nutritional aspects are under control, sequelae or end effects of all these stages should be followed as the child grows older.

Slow Motor Development

The group of VLBW babies (under 1000 g or 2 lb) are slow in motor development. They are slow in sitting, standing, and walking. These infants are evaluated with deductions made from their chronological age based on their gestational age at birth. For example, if the baby was born at 30 weeks of gestation, it was born 10 weeks before term (term pregnancy is 38 to 42 weeks, for an average of 40 weeks). Therefore, if the baby is evaluated at the age of 3 months in a follow-up visit, we deduct 10 weeks from 3 months. Thus, the baby is assessed as if he were 3 weeks old, and his neuromotor performance is compared to a 3-week norm and not a 3-month standard.

Physical Measurements

Weight, height, and head circumference are indices of great importance in evaluating the progress of these babies, particularly head circumference; by measuring head circumference, the pediatrician in the follow-up clinic is able to detect changes in the process of brain development (e.g., microcephaly, hydrocephaly).

The First Year

During the first year, the following problems may become apparent:

1. Deficits in motor development: muscle tone can be diminished or increased.
2. Vision problems, cataracts, glaucoma, or congenital anomalies involving vision.
3. Deafness.
4. Anomalies in head growth.

5. Seizure disorders resulting from brain damage at birth.

Evaluation of the High-Risk Premature Infant from the First to the Fifth Year of Age

During this period, deficits are reflected by the following signs:

1. Minor deficits in walking and motor coordination.
2. Language defects: expression, dyslexia, and comprehension.
3. Vision and hearing: myopia, strabismus (crossed eyes), and hearing deficits.
4. Behavior problems.
5. Hyperactivity.
6. Elements that identify the child with minimal brain dysfunction.

Tests Used to Evaluate the Child with Developmental Delay

1. Denver test. This test is ideal to document children with developmental delay in motor, social, and language areas.
2. Bayley test. This test is indicated to evaluate progress in development and maturation in a child between 6 months and 2 years of age.
3. Stanford–Binet test. This test evaluates intellectual potentials in a 3-year-old child.
4. Beery test. This test evaluates visual–motor integration at 4 years of age.

5. Zimmerman test. This test evaluates expression and language in specific learning problems.

Clinics for Follow-up of High-Risk Children

Hospitals that provide care for high-risk babies (intensive care units or perinatology centers) also have follow-up clinics for premature infants or high-risk infants where a group of specialists offer the benefit of care to these children as they grow up. They are trained in evaluating these infants to detect deficits early and to provide early treatment. Pediatricians, neonatologists, neurologists, pediatric physical therapists, orthopedists, nutritionists, ophthalmologists, and psychologists work together with the facilities of special laboratories (genetics, immunology, hematology, chemistry) as well as centers for special education and social services to offer the best standards of care in the process of rehabilitation of these children.

21

Seizures

Seizures may be an expression of central nervous system damage caused by asphyxial stress at birth. However, they could also be the only sequelae occurring later in life from a period of mild asphyxia that affected the baby during the perinatal stage.

There are four important elements in the evaluation of seizures in a newborn:

1. Mother's history.
2. Physical examination of the newborn with seizures.
3. Causes of seizures in the newborn.
4. Types of seizures or clinical forms.

Newborn seizures are involuntary movements affecting groups of muscles that may be generalized, with or without loss of consciousness; they are an expression of CNS dysfunction. The cause can be asphyxia, hemorrhage, trauma, metabolic disorder, or infectious disease, or they can be associated with congenital anomalies or inborn errors of metabolism.

Mother's History

It is very important to have a detailed history of the mother, a preliminary protocol covering the mother's past history, pregnancy, and type of delivery, in order to understand the causes or etiology of the newborn seizures.

For example, a history is needed of infections that may have affected the mother during pregnancy or at the time of delivery. In the case of intrauterine infections affecting a baby who at birth is small for gestational age (SGA) or an example of intrauterine growth retardation (IUGR), it is important to consider intrauterine viral infections, for example those caused by toxoplasmosis, rubella, cytomegalovirus, or herpes (TORCH). TORCH antibody titers should be requested in this group of SGA or IUGR newborn babies, who may be affected by any of these intrauterine viral infections. Intrauterine infections may explain, by infectious stress, the condition of small babies at birth with CNS involvement who are susceptible to seizures.

In newborn babies adequate for gestational age (AGA), seizures may also be an expression of infection, but here the infection is acquired at birth or shortly before or immediately after. These are examples of gram-negative bacterial infections acquired by the newborn at the time of delivery in spontaneous deliveries in cases of premature rupture of membranes (PROM) for more than 24 hr. This represents a bacterial infection affecting the urinary tract of the mother, for example, *E. coli, Proteus,* or *β-Streptococcus* responsible for the newborn sepsis with meningitis.

Metabolic factors as the cause of newborn seizures include the example of a newborn offspring of a diabetic mother, who is exposed to risk of hypoglycemia, which can cause seizures in the newborn baby large for gestational age (LGA). This could be diabetes class A, detected during pregnancy, or types B, C, or D in prospective mothers with a history of diabetes before pregnancy whether or not treated with insulin.

Systemic causes include cardiovascular causes, mothers with elevated blood pressure, and mothers with toxemia in whom a placental dysfunction causes hypertension, edema, and proteinuria in the mother and possibly results in complications such as eclampsia or seizures in the mother. This causes severe asphyxial risk in the fetus or newborn or severe depression in the newborn whose mother required treatment of this condition with $MgSO_4$, hypotensive drugs, and anticonvulsive medication.

Drugs are associated with convulsions in the newborn. Mothers of such infants may be using drugs or may be alcoholic, producing the so-called fetal alcohol syndrome in the newborn. This baby may present respiratory symptoms at birth, showing abnormalities in the face, heart, and joints. Seizures may complicate this condition and lead to mental retardation in later life.

Offspring of a mother who smokes more than 20 cigarettes a day during pregnancy may be SGA at birth and may have seizures as a result of ischemia or hypoxia of the brain created by nicotine.

It is also very important to evaluate the type of delivery by taking a detailed history of the mother. Deliveries represent an essential period in the life of the baby to be; exposure to trauma, asphyxia, and infection may leave the baby with the risk of seizures. Deliveries such as low forceps, breech, or vacuum may be traumatic for the baby, as can be cesarean section, which nevertheless may be a life-saving procedure for babies who are under the stress of prolonged labor. Also included are prolonged labor caused by dystocia or cephalopelvic disproportion (CPD), anomalies of contraction, and babies under risk of asphyxia because of placenta previa or abruptio placenta. These are situations that create trauma, asphyxia, and/or bleeding and can lead to seizures in the newborn.

Types of anesthesia given to the mother—general, spinal, or epidural—may affect the baby by leading to sedation or hypotension and by causing shock in the mother or the baby.

A cause of contamination at birth may be PROM for more than 24 hr in spontaneous vaginal deliveries. Sepsis and meningitis as complications of this type of delivery may lead to newborn seizures.

Acute bleeding caused by placenta previa or abruptio placenta is an obstetric emergency causing severe hemorrhage in the mother and acute anemia, hypotension, shock, and seizures in the newborn.

These are some of the facts in the mother's history that are essential for proper evaluation of the newborn with seizures.

Physical Examination of the Newborn with Seizures

It is very important to know the anthropometric values of the baby at birth, e.g., weight, height, and head circumference. These together with the elements of gestational assessment (skin, ears, areola, appearance of the external genitalia, and palmar and plantar creases) are essential findings in evaluating the degree of maturity of a newborn who develops seizures. Also significant is the presence of dysmorphic features representing either chromosomal (different trisomies) or congenital anomalies. This will allow the pediatrician to evaluate the maturity of the infant: term (38–42 weeks of gestation), preterm (less than 38 weeks of gestation), postterm (more than 42 weeks of gestation), a preterm baby who is SGA, or a case of IUGR.

This evaluation helps the pediatrician or neonatalogist to categorize the baby and to identify the different types of seizures affecting these groups. For example, in a term baby AGA by gestational assessment, the most frequent causes of seizures are trauma, asphyxia, fetal distress, aspiration of amniotic fluid (syndrome of meconium aspiration), oversedation, and anesthesia in the mother. These factors cause not only seizures but also infections because of PROM in the newborn.

If the baby is a preterm or SGA, seizures may be related to intrauterine factors, for example, intrauterine viral infections with CMV, rubella, herpes, or toxoplasmosis, explaining the positive TORCH antibody titers.

In the group of LGA babies, the most frequent cause of seizures is hypoglycemia or a metabolic factor and trauma because of the size of the baby. This would explain CPD which cause trauma and asphyxia in prolonged deliveries.

In very-low-birth-weight (VLBW) babies, seizures represent an expression of asphyxia and hemorrhage secondary to immaturity of major systems, particularly the brain and lungs, as well as to congenital anomalies that can be associated with birth size.

These findings in a physical examination represent the different categories of newborn babies and the specific types of seizures in each group (see Table 10).

In the physical examination of the newborn with seizures, these factors must be considered:

1. In a newborn baby with severe anemia, bleeding and hemolytic disease are possible etiologies.
2. A cyanotic baby without respiratory problems who has seizures at birth may be a possible case of congenital heart disease with cyanosis.
3. In the baby who is deeply jaundiced at birth, consider hemolytic disease with Rh or ABO incompatibility.
4. Infection must be entertained as a cause if it is known that the mother is febrile prior to or at delivery.

Clinical Forms of Newborn Seizures

Seizures in the newborn can be diagnosed as being of the following types:

1. Tonic.
2. Focal or clonic: jerking movements.
3. Myoclonic: rapid and slow movements combined.

Tonic seizures are expressed as rigidity in flexion or extension in either the neck or extremities. The EEG will show high-voltage and δ low waves.

Focal or clonic seizures have a pattern of shaking or jerking movements, observed mostly in the newborn with metabolic problems. An example is a newborn with hypoglycemia. In this type of seizure, the EEG will show high waves and spike activity.

Myoclonic seizures are described as frequent, repetitive, rapid, low-amplitude movements without control.

They present ocular changes. In this type of seizure the EEG shows a burst of suppression pattern.

Duration and degree of recovery are important elements for prognosis, as is the postictal status. In this postictal stage, the presence or absence of normal reflexes is important. If spontaneous movements return and the newborn reflexes such as grasp, Moro, tonic neck, and rooting are present without residual signs such as paresis, then the vital signs will be stable, and the prognosis is clinically favorable.

Prolonged apnea can be observed during the seizure stage, although apnea and bradycardia are not often seen in seizures. Apnea and hypoxia, if prolonged, explain color changes and cyanosis in the newborn.

In summary, hypoxia and ischemia are major causes of seizures, particularly in VLBW babies complicated by bleeding of different types; here the clinical symptoms are related to location of the hemorrhage in the brain matter.

In the term baby, asphyxia and ischemia caused by fetal distress may cause subcortical and subdural hemorrhage. Metabolic changes are observed in brain hemorrhage, including metabolic acidosis, hypocalcemia, and hypoglycemia.

In the LGA, expression of maternal diabetes (hypoglycemia and trauma) is a major cause of seizures.

Work-up in Seizures

In metabolic seizures, the work-up should include sugar and calcium blood levels; electrolytes (Na^+, Cl^-, K^+, HCO_3^-) are important to rule out metabolic acidosis.

In focal or clonic seizures associated with respiratory problems, a chest X ray should be obtained to rule out hyaline membrane disease (HMD), which has a characteristic pattern of granularity on air bronchogram.

In the postterm or postmature infant showing *in utero* signs of fetal distress (fetal bradycardia) indicating asphyxia *in utero* (which causes meconium aspiration syndrome), fetal asphyxia is associated with respiratory and metabolic acidosis. Such acidosis aggravates the prognosis of seizures in the postmature who suffered birth asphyxia.

In seizures related to infections (sepsis in the newborn), the work-up includes CSF for cultures and sensitivity. In infections present in the newborn representing SGA or IUGR, TORCH titers are indicated to rule out toxoplasmosis, rubella, cytomegalic disease, and herpes.

The hematologic work-up in the newborn with severe anemia or bleeding tendencies should include CBC, differential, platelet count, reticulocyte count, PT, and PTT.

The neurological work-up should include skull X ray to rule out calcification, sonogram and CAT scan to rule out CNS pathology and intracranial bleeding, as well as congenital anomalies or hydrocephalus, and CSF for cells, chemistry, and bacteriology.

Treatment of the Newborn with Seizures

The treatment will depend on the cause. In seizures related to metabolic problems such as hypoglycemia, the treatment aims to correct the hypoglycemia by giving intravenous 10 to 25% glucose at 2 or 3 ml/kg.

If seizures are related to low calcium, the treatment is 10% calcium gluconate at 2 ml/kg with monitoring of pulse or ECG.

In pyridoxine deficiencies the correction is with pyridoxine doses of 25–50 mg intravenously.

In status epilepticus (tonic–clonic seizures) treatment is with diazepam, 0.1–0.2 mg/kg intravenously.

22

Apnea and Sudden Infant Death Syndrome

Apnea

Apnea represents an episode of respiratory arrest or a pause in respiration. Pathological apnea is a period of lack of breathing that lasts 15 sec or more and is associated with slow heart rate (bradycardia) of 100/min or less. The concepts of apnea and bradycardia may vary: an example of bradycardia in a newborn is a pulse of 100 or less; bradycardia in an infant, associated with apnea, is a pulse less than 80; bradycardia of 40 associated with apnea is a severe bradycardia in an older child.

Apnea can be either central, with no respiratory effort, or peripheral, with respiratory effort. In central apnea, the cause involves CNS (respiratory center) damage because of anoxia, ischemia, or bleeding of the CNS in the small newborn. Other causes could be infection or metabolic or toxic factors. Peripheral apnea is caused by respiratory obstruction, either in the upper airway (newborn secretions) or in the lower lungs as a result of aspiration or RDS with immature lungs (HMD). Apnea may also be an expression of combined pathology, i.e., central and peripheral combined. For example, peripheral apnea in the premature newborn with HMD causing RDS initially leads to poor exchange as a result of hypoventilation and to systemic hypoxia of major organs such as the CNS. This will cause depression of the respiratory center and/or hypoxia and ischemia. Finally, the originally peripheral apnea complicated by central apnea may cause respiratory center depression.

There is a group of small premature babies with repeated episodes of apnea who are susceptible to near-miss sudden infant death syndrome (SIDS) and who, after passing the acute stage complicated with intraventricular hemorrhage (IVH) and metabolic and infectious factors, develop periods of apnea and bradycardia (A&B) after and during feedings. Here the etiology of A&B is presumably CNS, and it may be an expression of depression of the respiratory center or of peripheral chemoreceptor reactions to hypoxia or hypercapnia.

Etiology in Newborn Infants

1. CNS: bleeding, hypoxia (central apnea).
2. CV: CHD, PFC, BPD (peripheral apnea).
3. Infection: sepsis of the newborn with meningitis.
4. Metabolic: glucose, Ca^{2+}, PO_2, Na^+, HCO_3 (low levels).
5. Gastrointestinal.
6. Respiratory: HMD, meconium aspiration, bronchopulmonary dysplasia (BPD), atelectasis, pneumothorax.

Physiopathology

Central apnea involves the respiratory center, the brainstem, and the carotid body. Central apnea (CA) has been related to near-miss SIDS. Infants with prolonged "sleep apnea" or periodic breathing may reflect abnormalities in the central control of respiration (neurological control).

Different investigations have been carried out to determine response or failure in hypoxic arousal. Van Der Hal and co-workers (1985) have shown that failure to present hypoxic arousal may represent lack of chemoreceptor reactions to hypoxia or hypercapnia or depression of the respiratory center.

The Ondine syndrome or central congenital hypoventilation syndrome may represent a group of infants who fail to respond to 11% oxygen during sleep; without arousal response, this group of infants may be labeled as examples of failure of automatic control of respiration.

Sudden Infant Death Syndrome

Sudden infant death syndrome refers to the unexpected death of an infant under 1 year of age (usually under 6 months) with no previous history of disease and without specific necropsy findings. In the United States it is the cause of about 8000 deaths per year.

Possibly related etiologies include high-risk pregnancies with intrauterine infections (TORCH), nutritional deficits, alcohol or drug use, and systemic causes such as maternal hypertension or eclampsia and maternal infections such as UTIs. Other babies may be at high risk if they are premature, SGA, IUGR, or VLBW.

In the acute stage, i.e., the perinatal period (first 7 days), babies with IVH, HMD, infection (sepsis), jaundice (hyperbilirubinemia), and metabolic problems (hypoglycemia, hypocalcemia, acidosis) are especially susceptible to SIDS.

In the postacute stage, the neonatal period, SIDS is associated with episodes of A&B and with central or peripheral apneas.

Late-stage SIDS refers to sudden death occurring within the first 6 months of life.

23

The Future of the Hypoxic Child

For the newborn infant who starts life under significant hypoxic asphyxial stress, survival in the acute stage will depend on the nature of the insult and the type of care. For the newborn with minor asphyxial compromise, life prognosis may not be so threatening, but the child's future and his potentials as well as limitations will only become apparent as the child grows and develops.

The Child with Learning Disabilities

It is important to complete this volume with a review of the child with learning disabilities or minimal brain dysfunction. It should be emphasized that prenatal care, a normal delivery, the evaluation of pregnancies with problems, and early diagnosis and treatment will largely contribute to a healthy new life. The message is that a normal birth may be the main and most important factor for beginning a normal life.

169

It has been proved that the lack of oxygen at birth, birth asphyxia, causes significant problems in the process of delivery, and in the respiratory adjustment of a newborn going through a protracted labor and delivery. The depressed blue or cyanotic baby who does not respond with normal vitality, but who is treated in a medical center with all the proper facilities, is resuscitated in an intensive care unit, and recovers, may exhibit adverse consequences as he grows older.

If the stage of asphyxia at birth is severe, the child will show delayed motor development such as different types of paresis presenting cerebral palsy, the spastic type of hemiparesis, or diplegias.

In cases of less asphyxial compromise at birth, the child as he grows older may show moderate delay in motor development, both gross and fine, as well as delay in social habits and linguistic potentials. The child may be walking after 14 months, but sometimes motor development will be unaffected, occasionally with later speech impairment or different types of speech disorders or dyslexias.

Another sequela of birth asphyxia or difficult deliveries may bypass gross motor or language delays but show up as a child with hyperactive behavior (hyperkinetic), or a child with learning disabilities not because of low I.Q. but because excessive activity interferes with his concentration and attention span. His scholastic level will therefore be poor.

In general, the pediatrician taking the history of a child with learning disabilities will obtain a record of birth and pregnancy, investigating all the factors that may have affected pregnancy, including stages of delivery, weight progress, infections early in pregnancy, urinary tract infections, bleeding, anemias, hypertension in the mother, or history of diabetes. All these factors affect pregnancy and can create high-risk babies.

The type of delivery, term of pregnancy, and size of the baby all relate to the risk of trauma owing to breech, forceps, or prolonged deliveries with a risk of asphyxia and infection. All these factors may create fetal distress and interfere with healthy development later in life, but emphasis is given to asphyxial stress at birth, which, if prolonged, may cause bleeding associated with metabolic disorders or infections that would totally compromise the resistance of the newborn and lead to his future limitations.

From serious asphyxial stress at birth leading to a brain lesion, cerebral palsy, and serious deficits in motor, speech, and intellectual areas of expression to the child with minimal brain dysfunction, there are sequelae of all varieties. Thus, a multitude of defects may appear in later life.

If a history of birth trauma, brain stress from asphyxia complicated by metabolic or bleeding risks, and infection are ruled out, and the birth history is normal, then the child with a brain dysfunction or learning disability must have other causes or other factors to explain the syndrome. Infections during infancy and childhood, head trauma, familial diseases involving the central nervous system, genetic familial disorders, chromosomal dysfunctions, and metabolic or endocrine disorders may all create risks of future limitations in the child's development.

Again, the absence of all these causes and a normal condition at birth provide the best possible conditions for normal growth and development in motor, language, and intellectual skills. The prophylaxis for a healthy child is therefore summarized by recommending the following:

1. Early prenatal care and follow-up through pregnancy.
2. Diagnosis and treatment of high-risk pregnancies.
3. Deliveries in medical centers with facilities for tertiary care in cases of high-risk pregnancies and for delivering high-risk babies (neonatal ICU, perinatology centers). This will be the best contribution to family planning to assure having a healthy child.

Early Diagnosis of Minimal Brain Dysfunction

This usually takes place in the preschool years because the child's milestones up to preschool age may have been normal. The minimal brain dysfunction (MBD) child may have average, high, or low intelligence but may fail to show good academic achievement because of behavioral differences in relationships with teachers and peers. Characteristics of the MBD child include:

1. Inability to learn.
2. Deficit of attention span.
3. Deficit in receptive, integrative, or expressive language.
4. Deficit in memory.
5. Aberration in motor activity.
6. Deficit in coordination.
7. Deficit in perception, auditory and visual.
8. Deficit in comprehension, abstraction, and organization of different levels.

TABLE 18. The Future of the Hypoxic or Asphyxiated Child

	Hypoxia (clumsy child)	Asphyxia (cerebral palsy)
Etiology	Minimal birth injury Hypoxia *in utero* or perinatal Apgar 5–7	Severe asphyxia *in utero* or perinatal Apgar <5
Other intrauterine factors	Systemic disease Nutrition Infection Drugs, alcohol	Same
Motor	Low tone Clumsy Ataxic or athetoid Hyperreflexia	Spastic Hypertonicity Hyperreflexia, clonus Increased tone
Head circumference	Normal	Microcephalic
Intellectual	Normal to low I.Q. Normal to low verbal performance MBD behavior: poor concentration, overactive, learning disorder	Severe deficit Very low I.Q. Retarded verbal performance Dyslexia
Physical performance as an older child	Poor Careless, poor writing Falls easily Slow in athletic activities	Paresis may improve after 1–2 years Severe spasticity may cause deformities
Joints	Hyperextensible	Stiff, limited range Spastic arthropathy Muscle spasm

9. Lability of emotions.
10. Impulsiveness.

It should be emphasized that the MBD child or the child with specific learning disability is not a retarded child (child with a low I.Q.). The MBD child may have one or more of the deficits mentioned above but have average or above average intelligence. Consequently, in school he should be managed differently and separately from regular class children and from retarded children.

The Mixed Minimal Brain Dysfunction

The majority of MBD children belong to the mixed-MBD group. The most common is a child with language deficit manifested by (1) reading and spelling difficulties, (2) short attention span, and (3) mild to moderate hyperactivity.

Moderate to Severe Asphyxia

Moderate to severe asphyxia may lead in later life to clumsiness or cerebral palsy (see Table 18).

24

Perinatology Goals

Over the last two decades great improvement has been made in prophylaxis and treatment of the high-risk pregnancy, resulting in high-risk infants who present with very low birth weight, as small for gestational age, or showing intrauterine growth retardation.

Fetal monitoring, developed by Caldeyro-Barcia as a way to detect fetal asphyxia and prevent it, was and is a great contribution to the well-being of the present generation and future generations.

Significant progress has been made in perinatology in the diagnosis of a group of babies who, because of their constitution, will face major stress during labor. These babies may be identified by new techniques such as amniocentesis, fetal monitoring, and sonography, and research on fetal breathing movements is promising.

Much progress has been made in offering the high-risk infant the best environment in which to survive the birth period, in tertiary centers where the technology, equipment, and personnel are available to overcome the risks of the perinatal period.

175

The challenge at present is the identification of the high-risk infant and the management of this type of infant to minimize or prevent the sequelae.

Heart, lung, kidneys, and liver are organs that survive the risks of perinatal asphyxia without residual effects; thus, the major threat is brain asphyxia and brain hemorrhage as causes of death or neurological sequelae. The sequelae of cerebral palsy, minimal brain dysfunction, and seizure disorders offer the incentive for early detection of these abnormalities in order to give the best results with rehabilitation and to offer a better life. The challenge is clear. The progress so far is remarkable, but it is not yet complete. This is an invitation to work together to make this goal a reality.

Bibliography

Auld PAM: Respiratory distress syndrome of the newborn, in Scarpelli EM, Auld PAM, and Goldman MS (eds): *Pulmonary Diseases of Fetus and Newborn and Child*. Philadelphia, Lea & Febiger, 1978, pp 447–518.

Behrman IS: Obstetrical management of prematurity, in Fanaroff AA, Martin RJ (eds): *Neonatal and Perinatal Medicine: Diseases of the Fetus and Infant*, ed. 3. St. Louis, C.V. Mosby, 1983, pp 133–196.

Bertan M: Strategies for the at risk fetus infant. Child Health 1984;3:125–136.

Bhat R, Raju TNK, Vidyasagar D: Immediate and long term outcome of infants less than 1,000 grams. *Crit Care Med* 1978;6:147–150.

Blumenthal Bash D, Gold WA: *The Nurse and the Child-Bearing Family*. New York, Wiley, 1981, pp 567–663.

Boddy K, Dawes GS: Fetal well-being and fetal breathing, in Turnbull AC, Woodford FP (eds): *Prevention of Handicap through Antenatal Care*. New York, Elsevier, 1976, pp 123–125.

Bolognese RJ, Schwarz RH, Schneider J (eds): *Perinatal Medicine*, ed 2. Baltimore, Williams & Wilkins, 1982, pp 223–243.

Caldeyro-Barcia R: Physiology of fetal circulation, in Cassels DE (ed): *The Heart and Circulation in the Newborn Infant*. New York, Grune & Stratton, 1966, pp 7–36.

Caldeyro-Barcia R: Obstetrical interference. *Birth Family J* 1975;2:34–38.

Dan M, Levine SZ, New EV: The development of prematurely born children with birth weights or minimal postnatal weights of 1,000 grams or less. *Pediatrics* 1958;22:1037–1052.

Dweck HS, Saxon SA, Benton JW, Cassady G: Early development of the tiny premature infant. *Am J Dis Child* 1973;126:28–34.

Feldman S: *Choices in Childbirth*. New York, Grosset & Dunlap, 1979, pp 52–59.

Fitzhardinge PM: Early growth and development in low birthweight infants following treatment in an intensive care nursery. *Pediatrics* 1975;56:162–172.

Fitzhardinge PM: Follow-up studies in infants treated by mechanical ventilation. *Clin Perinatol* 1978;5:451–459.

Francis-Williams J, Davies P: Very low birthweight and later intelligence. *Dev Med Child Neurol* 1974;16:709–728.

Fuchs F: Prevention of perinatal diseases and injuries. *Child Health* 1984;3:65–89.

Gasser RF: *Atlas of Human Embryology*. Hagerstown, MD, Harper & Row, 1975, pp 25–297.

Goodlin RC: *Care of the Fetus*. Paris, Masson, 1979, pp 221–254.

Holmes DL, Reigh JN, Pasternak J: *The High Risk Infant Beyond the Neonatal Period*. Hillsdale, NJ, Lawrence Erlbaum, 1984, pp 126–149.

Illingworth R: *Basic Developmental Screening, 0–2 Years.* Oxford, Blackwell, 1977.

Jensen K: *Reproduction: The Cycle of Life.* Washington, US Newsbooks, 1982, pp 71–81.

Kelly DH, Shannon D: Neonatal and infantile apnea, in Milunsky A, Friedman EA, Gluck L (eds): *Advances in Perinatal Medicine,* vol 1. New York, Plenum Medical, 1981, pp 1–44.

Kuman SP, Ankay EK, Sacks LM, et al: Follow-up studies of very low weight infants (1200 g or less) born and treated at the perinatal center. *Pediatrics* 1980;66:438–444.

Lee K, Paneth N, Gartner LM, et al: Neonatal mortality: An analysis of the recent improvement in the United States. *Am J Public Health* 1980;70:15–21.

Little WJ: On the influence of abnormal parturition, difficult labours, premature birth, and asphyxia neonatorum on the mental and physical condition of the child, especially in relation to deformities. *Trans Obstet Soc Lond* 1861–1862;3:293–344.

Lubchenco LO, Horner FA, Reed LH, et al: Sequelae of premature birth. *Am J Dis Child* 1963;106:135–149.

Maloney J, Brodecky V, Wilkinson M, Walker A: Placental insufficiency and the development of the respiratory system in utero, in Tildon JT (ed): *SIDS.* New York, Academic Press, 1983, pp 305–318.

Milliez JM, James S: Fetal Physiology, in Aladjem S, Brown AK, Sureau C (eds): *Clinical Perinatology.* St Louis, CV Mosby, 1980, pp 52–67.

Moore K: *The Developing Human.* Philadelphia, WB Saunders, 1977, pp 12–140.

Moore ML: *Realities in Childbearing.* Philadelphia, WB Saunders, 1983, pp 439–598.

National Center for Health Statistics: *Vital Statistics of the*

US 1967, vol 1: *Natality*. Washington, US Department of Health, Education and Welfare (PHS), 1970.

National Center for Health Statistics: *Vital Statistics of the US 1975*, vol 1: *Natality*. Washington, US Department of Health, Education and Welfare (PHS), 1978.

Pansky B: *Review of Medical Embryology*. New York, Macmillan, 1982, pp 44–110.

Pape KE, Fitzhardinge P: Perinatal damage to the developing brain, in Milunsky A, Friedman EA, Gluck L (eds): *Advances in Perinatal Medicine*, vol 1. New York, Plenum Medical, 1981, pp 45–85.

Pilliteri A: *Maternal Newborn*. Boston, Little Brown, 1981, pp 145–181.

Read DJC: Many paths to asphyxial deaths, in Tildon JT (ed): *SIDS*. New York, Academic Press, 1983, pp 183–196.

Rugh R, Shettles LB: *From Conception to Birth*. New York, Harper & Row, 1971.

Rumack CM, Johnson ML: Perinatal and infant brain imaging, in Perveiler FM (ed): *Intracranial Hemorrhage: Role of Ultrasound and Computed Tomography*, Chicago, Year Book, 1984, pp 117–147.

Saigal S, Rosenbaum P, Stoskopf B, Milner R: Follow-up of infants 501 to 1500 gm birthweight delivered to residents of a geographically defined region with perinatal intensive care facilities. *J Pediatr* 1982;100:606–613.

Spitzer AR, Fox WW: The use and abuse of mechanical ventilation, in Stern L (ed): *Hyaline Membrane Disease*. New York, Grune & Stratton, 1984, pp 145–173.

Stewart AL, Turcan DM, Rawlings G, et al: Prognosis for infants weighing 1000 grams or less at birth. *Arch Dis Child* 1977;52:97–104.

Tucker S: *Fetal Monitoring.* St. Louis, CV Mosby, 1978, pp 73–139.

Van Der Hal AL, Rodriguez AM, Sergent CW, Platzke AC: Hypoxic and hypercapnic arousal responses and prediction of subsequent apnea in infancy. *Pediatrics,* May 1985, pp 848–854.

Voorhies T, Vanucci R: Perinatal neurology, in Boyd R, Battaglia F (eds): *Perinatal Medicine.* London, Butterworths, 1983, pp 70–112.

Index